Cracked Marbles
Life's Lessons for a Maine Surgeon

Tom Palmer, MD

Tiffin Press of Maine

Cracked Marbles
Life's Lessons for a Maine Surgeon

Published by: TIFFIN PRESS OF MAINE
110 Jones Point Road
Brooksville, Maine 04617
www.tiffinpress.com

Senior Editor: Joan MacCracken, MD, Brooksville, Maine
Assistant Editor: Joan M Holmberg
Cover Photo: Susan Jenkins-Urban, Sedgwick, Maine
Interior illustration: Molly O Holmberg
Design Consultant: David Fickett,
Downeast Graphics, Ellsworth, Maine

Note to Reader: This book recounts the essence of my experience. The book
is not intended to be a literal account, and all names and specific details of the
patients and physicians are fiction based on fact and should not to be taken as
a portrayal of any living person.

Acknowledgement is made for permission to reprint
"The Art and Science of Medical Care" by Tom Palmer, MD, first published
in Op-Ed piece in *Bangor Daily News* on February 23, 2002.

Library of Congress Control Number   2008901628
Library of Congress Cataloging-in-Publication Data
Palmer, Tom, MD (1924-   )
Cracked Marbles: Life's Lessons for a Maine Surgeon
1. Medicine---Maine---Anecdotes   2. Medicine, Rural—Maine---Bangor
3. Surgery----Maine

ISBN# 978-09646018-8-8

*to my patients who entrusted me
with their health and lives
and became my friends*

A special thanks....

    for the guiding inspiration of the late Robin Crabtree Haskell, who stimulated my interest in writing and encouraged me to pick up the pen,
    for Ardeana Hamlin, our published Bangor author, and Meg Haskell, journalist and former nurse, who both encouraged me as well,
    for the late Nancy Bach and her husband, Dr. Robert Bach, who advised me to just put something down on paper and the rest would follow,
    for my late wife Mary Ellen and children, Tom, Ed, Anne, David, and Jim, who supported me throughout my many years of taking care of other people,
    and finally, my gratitude goes to my editor, Dr. Joan MacCracken, my catalyst and inspiration, without whom this book would not have been published.

                                                Tom

Contents

Foreword

Medicine was good for Tom Palmer and Tom Palmer was good for medicine. His life has been one dedicated to helping others. He stood tall in the arena of medical care during a period when the relationship of patient and physician was prized, when physicians were colleagues, there to help each other. As a highly respected general surgeon in Bangor for thirty-five years, Tom provided many with a stellar example of what a physician could be. Dr. Palmer insists that he learned valuable lessons from his patients, lessons that he would carry through his entire life.

I had the privilege of working in association with Tom in surgery practice for seven years. He soon became an inspiration and a mentor. When he signed out a patient for his weekend off, he always referred to them by name, followed by a little personal clip about them. You never heard him say, "There is a gallbladder in room 308 who can be discharged in the morning." It would be something like, "Mrs. Jones in room 308 can go home tomorrow and by the way, her father was the first sheriff of Piscataquis County." Tom never complained about being called to the Emergency room, no matter what the hour, for his philosophy was that "it was a privilege to practice medicine and help other human beings." I often repeated that phrase on my trips into the ER in the wee hours of the morning, and it bore fruits of a friendly greeting to the anxious patient who awaited me.

After preparing at Harvard College and then at Tufts University Medical School, he completed a rotating internship, two years in the Navy, and a general surgical residency at New England Medical Center. In 1956 Tom decided to move to Bangor with his wife Mary Ellen, a Bangor native, and begin his general surgical practice at Eastern Maine General. Initially, the general practitioners, who were performing general surgery, tried to discourage him from coming. At first, few patients came his way, but after saving the life of an osteopathic doctor from a gunshot wound in the chest and abdomen, people took note of his skill and began sending patients to him.

Over the years Dr. Palmer became a leader in Maine medicine in addition to being a dedicated, compassionate surgeon. He was certified by the American Board of Surgery. Tom served as President of the Medical Staff at Eastern Maine Medical Center, Chief of Surgery at St. Joseph's Hospital, and President of the Maine Chapter of the American College of Surgeons. He was subsequently appointed to the Board of Directors of Eastern Maine Healthcare. Yet, in the hallways of the hospitals among the nurses, he was fondly known as "a true prince," and he always maintained his gentle manner.

Throughout his career he has maintained his sense of humor, his humble attitude, and his caring touch. That he has written these remarkable stories about his patients is no surprise. He has always been one to tell a good tale. Tom Palmer continues to give to others, to read extensively, and to follow the changes in medicine.

May these stories be a reminder to my younger colleagues that the personal touch in medicine is sacred and should never be overcome by the advancing wave of technology in our time.

Robert Bach, MD
North Haven, Maine

Preface

Many of us are familiar with the 1891 oil painting by Sir Luke Fildes "The Doctor" in which a desperately ill child lies with arm outstretched toward her physician who sits beside her, leaning forward with hand on his bearded chin. His intense gaze is fixed on the child as if willing his patient to get well with powerful vibrations. In the background is the shadowy figure of the child's father whose anxiety is etched upon his face. That doctor had painfully inadequate treatment to offer the little girl other than cold pack applications for fever reduction and drinks of fluid to maintain hydration, but his compassion, dedication, untiring devotion to his calling and respect for human life shine brightly from the lamplight of the canvas. He was clearly prepared to stay at that patient's side through the night if needed, waiting for the fever to subside and the crisis to pass. The painting reflects the wonderful art of the practice of medicine at a time when the science of medicine was sadly undeveloped.

As we all know, the science of medicine has wondrously been developed in the century since that painting was created. The doctor is now armed with a myriad of powerful weapons to combat and overcome disease and injury. The weapons include antibiotics, vaccines, drugs to control physical and mental illnesses, intravenous fluid, blood transfusion, chemotherapy, hemodialysis, anesthesia techniques which permit refined surgical operations, organ transplantation, to name only some. We now have marvelous and expensive diagnostic tools such as laboratory tests, x-rays, electrocardiography, sonography, angiography, computed axial tomography (CAT scans), magnetic resonance imagery (MRIs), laparoscopy, endoscopy and others that allow us to evaluate and peer inside almost every organ and nook and cranny of the human body.

Science has developed the amazing computer, which, unlike the human mind that actively forgets facts and knowledge, stores with infallible and retrievable memory all the information that is submitted to it. Machines can more efficiently manage the huge amount of scientific knowledge available for accurate diagnosis and treatment. However, medical care is slowly being depersonalized. Gradually, the physician is being replaced by the computer and by individuals with limited medical training. There is now the potential that the art of medical care will be relegated to history and replaced by cold science, which is a disturbing prospect. The computer has no feelings or emotions.

The human aspect of medical care is of greatest importance. Patients trust and confide in their physicians to whom they reveal their lives' most intimate aspects, fears and concerns. Patients require the emotional support, understanding, and compassion of a dedicated fellow human being, especially in life-threatening situations and at life's inevitable end. The most successful doctors (and those least often sued) are those who consider the patient to be their friend and not a business customer. Dr. Bernard Siegel, surgeon and author, in 1993 wrote, "This century began with people praying to be saved from diphtheria and will finish with people praying for heart transplants. Let us utilize and enjoy the benefits of science but not forget the human beings who are our patients. When I asked three very ill young patients what they wanted me to say at an oncology meeting, they said, "Tell them to treat me like a person. Tell them to let me talk first. Tell them to knock on my door, say hello and goodbye and look me in the eye when they talk to me."" (*Love, Medicine & Miracles*)

The warning signs that science and technology are gradually replacing the art in medical care are everywhere. A patient complained that in the visit to her physician, "The doctor sat in front of a computer and never looked away from the computer screen. There was no eye contact at all." Another patient stated that if he met his physician of three years on the street, he would not recognize him because technicians, nurses, and physician assistants always provided his medical care, allowing increased "productivity" for the practice. Yet another mentioned during her visit to the doctor that she had unexpectedly developed a new troublesome symptom. She was told to make another appointment for the new problem because her allotted time was used up. And sadly, a computer-generated letter from a doctor's office was addressed to a man who had died two and a half months earlier, only to remind him that he had not arranged for his annual flu shot and that it was important to his health. A hospital nurse found her patient sitting by the bedside weeping and distraught. The doctor had just told her that the tests showed a blockage in her coronary arteries and that a heart surgeon would come the next day to arrange an operation to correct this. The physician then turned on his heels and left the room without another word. The patient was devastated.

The house call by the physician has become a relic of the past. At the patient's home the doctor has none of his scientific tools available. Time-wise and economically, the house call was an inefficient practice. Today, it has evolved that many doctors never even leave their office and computer for patient care. He or she becomes less than a complete physician, a "doc in a box," so to speak. When a patient, whose doctor knows and understands him or her, becomes acutely ill, that patient is now sent off to physician strangers at the hospital (called hospitalists) who may or may not have access to the patient's life records. The original doctor loses contact with his patient and only after hospitalization receives a summary of the illness, diagnosis, treatment, and results. With each succeeding illness, another complete set of strangers may be the caregivers. This type of fragmented care may be perhaps inevitable in the future, and many young doctors seem to welcome it. The new system is good for the involved physicians who work regular, limited hour shifts. They don't become exhausted from the long, stressful days and nights on call. They have time for hobbies such as golf, fishing, skiing, and boating. Their marriages are not put at risk due to absence from or lack of participation in family activities. But, is it really better from the viewpoint of the patient who is the important person in all this? In an often-quoted lecture by Dr. Francis Peabody in 1926 entitled, "The Approach to the Patient," he stated, "The secret of caring for the patient is caring for the patient." This remains true more than three quarters of a century later. Science is certainly a necessity, technology, a valuable tool, but they should never replace the art of patient care.

It is my sincere hope that the following stories provide for the reader a glance backwards at the art of medicine, when there was time for the doctor/patient relationship to grow and blossom, when listening to and caring for another human being in need was the satisfying essence of doctoring. Through all my years of practice, I have learned from my patients who have taught me so much about life in its fullest measure. In the end it really is all about the people.

Tom Palmer, MD
Bangor, Maine 2008

The Beginnings

Harry Byrd was a sickly child. Severe asthma kept him from physical activities. Often, especially on damp cold days, when he went outside to play games with friends, he would soon be back in the house, wheezing and gasping for breath while inhaling steam over a teapot on the stove. Ipecac was a favorite home remedy in those days. It substituted one miserable situation with another. A swallowed teaspoon of the powerful emetic promptly produced nausea and forceful vomiting. This released the bronchial spasm and restored easy breathing. It was not very encouraging when young Harry overheard his mother telling her lady friends, "Some nights I stand at the foot of his bed while he struggles for air and pray that God will take him." Every germ that came along found him an easy victim. He had flu, measles, whooping cough, scarlet fever, tonsillitis, and ear abscesses among other things. Because of frequent forced absences, Harry Byrd had to repeat the third grade. He grew tall, but skinny and pale. Often adults looked at him appraisingly and asked, "When are you going to put on some weight?" Harry couldn't answer that, but he ate large amounts of food at every meal with no results. An aunt, who was known for attributing most illnesses to the thyroid gland, advised a metabolism test. This was done and was normal. Family visitors, especially his many aunts, looked him over critically, shook their heads sympathetically, and gave him unsolicited advice to plan for a nice easy job like school teaching because he would have all summers off. They were of the opinion that Harry would not live very long and told him so. He eventually learned that the aunts were not all that omniscient and that school teaching was not that easy, but actually a tough and demanding profession.

Because of this background Harry Byrd developed a deep and lasting sense of inferiority. He had close kinship and feelings of empathy with fellow humans who were impaired by illness, injury or birth defect. He wanted to do something to help others. Since he could not achieve physical prowess, he concentrated on developing and expanding his mind. He read everything he could from the school library-- history, fiction, Classics. At that time medical educators had become concerned that too much emphasis was being placed on science and not enough on the human aspects of the art of medical care. Byrd decided that he would be a medical doctor and chose the humanities for his major college emphasis with less concentration on chemistry, physics, and mathematics. Thus, the way was prepared to mold him into a people doctor rather than primarily a scientist.

Byrd was accepted to medical school and flourished there. He was fascinated by the new world of learning how to help sick people. The first two years of training in medical school were devoted to learning in great detail about the normal human body and the things that might go wrong with it. There were so many entities where human health could be derailed that Harry Byrd wondered how anyone escaped illness and abnormality for very long. Finally, at the end of the two year study, the future doctors were introduced to live fellow humans, known professionally as "patients," for reasons that were obscure.

Harry's group of four students were led as observers by a young operating room nurse into the sacrosanct operating room after they were carefully attired in cap, gown, mask, and shoe covers. The nurse warned them not to touch anything on or near the sterile instrument table and drapes. Harry Byrd listened with fascination as the surgeon explained what needed to be done to remove the diseased gallbladder of the man lying on the table before him. A swift movement of the scalpel across the patient's exposed abdomen was accompanied by a flow of bright red blood. Harry Byrd fainted dead away onto the floor. The next thing he remembered was the nurse peering down at him above her mask and her beautiful brown eyes laughing. He struggled to get up, but she pushed him gently back down and told him to just stay there for a bit. At that moment, if anyone told Byrd that he would spend his entire professional life as a surgeon, he would have pronounced that person undoubtedly insane.

On the next day Harry Byrd and a classmate met two patients at the outpatient clinic of a large teaching hospital. A young medical resident was their teacher. He wore immaculate, white trousers and jacket and carried an air of omniscience about him to the envy of his neophyte students. He explained their mission to interview and examine their first live patients.

The first was a friendly, smiling, elderly, grey-haired lady who walked into the examining room with a cane. She had the gnarled hands and wrists of a person with obvious arthritis. Harry Byrd asked her about her symptoms, the joints involved, the amount of disability, and the effect on her family situation. She lived in an apartment with her aged husband, who had multiple medical problems. She spoke with a distinct Irish brogue. Byrd looked at the medical record chart before him and apologized. He said he had been given the wrong patient's record, namely that of Sadie Goldstein, obviously a lady of different ethnicity.

"I am Sadie," she said, laughing. "I was born and raised in Dublin, Ireland. We have quite a few Jewish people there. As a matter of fact, the Lord Mayor of Dublin, Mr. Briscoe, God bless him, is Jewish."

Harry Byrd completed his examination and decided afterwards that he had learned more from the experience than just about arthritis.

The resident explained that the next patient had heart valve damage from childhood rheumatic fever. He described in detail the sh-lub-dub, lub-sh-dub of diastolic, systolic, and other audible murmurs and where on the chest wall each could best be heard with the stethoscope. Byrd and his student partner Leon went into the examination room.

The patient was age twenty, statuesque, naked from the waist up. She smiled happily at them over her shoulder as she sat on the examination table. Obviously, Byrd thought this young lady was not only proud of her heart murmurs, which had been listened to by the entire class of medical students, but also of her splendid physique which hadn't been exposed to the ravages of time. Harry Byrd first introduced himself to the young lady. Then, carefully, he listened as instructed for the sh-lub-dub and lub-sh-dub, while trying not to be distracted by the anatomic geography so close by. He thought he could hear the appropriate sounds and then stood back for his classmate to listen. Leon spent a considerable period of time listening with furrowed brow. All of a sudden Byrd realized to his horror that the ear pieces of Leon's stethoscope were around his neck and not in his ears at all. Finally, Leon stepped back, and the two students went back into the adjacent hall.

"Did you hear the murmurs?" Byrd asked.

"Oh yeah!" his partner responded enthusiastically. Harry again learned from this patient. He wondered if Leon had.

During the four years of medical school Harry's asthma disappeared. He stopped getting victimized by illness, and he began to gain weight. He enjoyed these years and excelled. At graduation he was surprised to learn that he had won honors and was now ready for his new life.

Harry Byrd had to choose a field of medicine to pursue for his future professional life and was inclined toward the various surgical fields despite his first discouraging experience in the operating room. He was accepted into an internship program at a large teaching hospital where he would have a broad experience in a variety of areas, namely general surgery, obstetrics and gynecology, orthopedic surgery, urology, anesthesiology, and emergency service.

At first, obstetrics seemed appealing. He thought that it was in general a happy field helping brand new citizens into the world, and in modern times rare deaths among the mothers and infants. However, that concept rapidly changed with experience. The labor and delivery process usually involved long nights and days. The patient care was routine, but when an emergency did occur, it was sudden, complex, and a threat to life. For example, the placenta, the vital connection between mother and unborn baby, could prematurely separate from the uterus, and threaten the life of the infant. Also, the placenta could by chance be improperly attached to the uterus and block the passage of the baby through the birth canal causing severe hemorrhage. Possible developmental abnormalities could be complex for the infant immediately or in the future.

Harry Byrd, the intern in obstetrics, was assigned, among other duties, to the night duty in the delivery room. He slept very little on a cot facing the doors of the two elevators that brought the mothers in labor to deliver the new citizen. He thought of the story of "The Tiger or the Lady" in which the early Christian prisoner was required to choose and open one of the two identical doors in the amphitheater. Behind one was a fierce and hungry tiger ready to attack him and behind the other was a beautiful, smiling, young woman waiting to greet him with open arms.

As he lay on his cot in the middle of one night, an elevator door opened and out came a young woman who was not smiling. She was in advanced labor and was without any prenatal studies or care. The patient was rushed off the elevator by attendants and directly onto a delivery table. Byrd's nurse associate put the woman's legs up in the stirrups, and then briefly left the room to get some warm blankets. Byrd sat down on a stool between the up-stretched legs, and almost immediately, the baby was delivered into his gloved hands. He placed the screaming newborn baby crosswise on the mother's lower abdomen between her thighs and reached around behind himself to get some instruments on the table there to prepare for the expulsion of the afterbirth. Suddenly, the baby lurched and fell off the mother's abdomen. Byrd turned back to see the baby screaming and red-faced in protest at being removed from the warm fluid environment inside his mother's uterus. The baby boy was swinging back and forth by the still attached umbilical cord like a pendulum over the wastebasket below. Byrd quickly replaced the baby on the mother just as the nurse reentered the room. The umbilical cord was cut and tied, the placenta removed, and the new citizen was wrapped in a warm blanket, which pacified him as he was placed in a crib. The only individuals who observed this misadventure were Harry Byrd and the newborn swinger, neither one of whom would inform anyone else. The mother, exhausted and relieved of the pain of her labor, had her eyes closed, and the nurse was out of the room.

On another occasion a few nights later, the elevator door again opened, and an obese, older woman was brought into the delivery area. She was in apparent advanced labor, with severe spasms of pain in the lower abdomen every few minutes. Harry Byrd asked appropriate questions. There had been no previous pregnancies, and no prenatal studies or care. She was forty-five and had never married. Her regular menstrual periods had stopped nine months previously. Byrd examined her large, round abdomen and percussed it, thumping with his fingers. There was no solid tissue immediately beneath the surface, only air. He listened to the abdomen with his stethoscope for fetal heart sounds. There were none. So Byrd sat down beside the woman. He told her that contrary to what she believed, she was not pregnant, but in view of her age and marital status that might not be so bad. He explained that she, like some other women before her, was afflicted by a false pregnancy, which is called by the elaborate term "Psuedocyesis." False pregnancy was not rare, but it usually didn't progress this far. He recommended that she have studies to be certain that other problems, like bowel obstruction, were not present to explain the abdominal distention. With that, the woman jumped off the examination table, demanded her clothes, and headed for the elevator after announcing in a loud voice that she was going to the Beth Israel Hospital where the doctors knew what they were doing. Harry Byrd decided that perhaps a different field of medicine might suit him better in his future.

In contrast, Byrd's emergency department experience was exciting, stimulating, and challenging, varying from simple to complex. He treated the straight forward, less complicated situations, like lacerations and some fractures, and he initiated studies that would lead to solving a diagnostic problem. But there was usually a single encounter with the patient and follow-up was difficult. The patient was either sent home, to his own doctor, or admitted into the hospital for ongoing studies and therapy.

One event during that rotation was permanently etched on Harry Byrd's mind and kept coming back to his consciousness at unexpected times. He was standing with a young nurse near the first floor stairwell in the emergency department. They were discussing the plan for a patient's care. Suddenly and silently a human being came down from above and crashed with a sickening thud on the floor between them. The person was dead on impact. Investigation of the horrifying event disclosed that this was a patient on the fifth floor surgery ward who had undergone multiple radical operations for extensive cancer of his mouth, jaw, and face. A large, deforming defect had resulted, and more reconstructive surgery was planned. Return of the cancer was a threat as well. The man had suffered agony, stress, and depression through this ordeal and had decided to end it all. He jumped over the railing and fell five stories to his relief by death. Harry Byrd thought about this man many times. What had the man's life been like? Did he have a wife, children whom he loved and loved him in return? What kind of work did he do? Could the cancer have been prevented? Did he chew tobacco or smoke too much? Did his doctors focus their attention entirely on the dread cancer and not on the fellow human being, the person afflicted? Under similar circumstances of physical torture and mental anguish, what would he, Harry, do himself? Perhaps, suicide appeared to the patient as the only way out of his problems. It was unclear what hospital authorities thought about this tragedy. They took a practical approach to the problem and installed heavy screening across the stairwell on each floor of the patient care building and in their wisdom put locks on all the windows.

He continued through the other fields of anesthesiology, urology, and orthopedics, but none of these appealed to him. His final assignment of his internship was general surgery. It proved to be the field to which he would devote his entire professional life. The great variety of problems which came to him for diagnosis and treatment were exciting and challenging. In the fields of general surgery, diseases of the head and neck, skin, breasts, lymph nodes, arteries, and veins were common, sometimes simple, but often difficult to diagnose as well as treat. The abdomen presented an entire field of complex and mysterious problems hidden behind muscular walls.

Byrd quickly realized that the diseases that he would deal with did not exist alone in a vacuum. Each one was like a stone dropped into a pond with concentric ripples radiating out from the center. Likewise, the illness or injury of a father or mother had great ramifications in the function and obligations of all the family members and had to be dealt with. Intimate knowledge of families was an important part of the patient's care.

The qualification for general surgery required at least four additional years of intensive, demanding training and experience after internship. Harry Byrd enthusiastically entered and engaged those difficult but fascinating years of residency training.

High Finances

Harry Byrd was uncertain whether he had made the right decision in moving to Maine after five long years of surgical training following medical school in Boston. After all, there were a dozen men doing surgery in this Maine city, and none of them had encouraged the neophyte to move north. However, only four of the twelve had completed formal training in surgery. Three others had some surgical training, and the rest had learned "on the job" with varying degrees of success. If the truth were known, two and probably three of them had so little knowledge and natural or acquired ability that they should never have lifted a scalpel. One easy way for Byrd to get started in his chosen field was to be the associate of a surgeon with an established practice, but no one invited him, and besides, he preferred to be independent.

So, it was not without a certain amount of apprehension that Byrd and his wife Avis made the move to Maine. After a few months in a rented apartment they decided to buy a house. They went to the bank on a bright spring morning to arrange a mortgage for their first home. The bank was a massive, square, granite building situated on the edge of the Kenduskeag Stream, which passed through the middle of town. The bank presented an imposing image of strength, just as its architects had intended.

As the couple went into the bank through its heavy oak doors, Byrd noticed a worker sandpapering a large patch of green paint from the front of the building. He knew that paint had been left there by Enos Whitworth, one of his patients in the hospital. Enos was a young man from Lincoln, a town about thirty miles to the north, and like many other young Maine people, he had moved south to Connecticut to find work in the Pratt and Whitney aircraft engine factory. But Enos had gotten lonesome and had decided to come home for a weekend with his friends and relatives. On Friday, after work on the three to eleven p.m. shift, he set out alone in his old green Chevy coupe with a pint of vodka on the seat beside him. Whenever he felt sleepy during the long night-time drive home, he took a couple of swigs from the bottle to stimulate himself, and that was a bad mistake. By the time he came into Bangor on Route 2 (Interstate 95 not yet having been extended north of Augusta), the bottle was empty. As dawn was breaking, Enos drove down the hill into town, heading on through to his destination in Lincoln. At the bottom of the hill he went straight into the granite front wall of the bank instead of veering left with the road. The bank was unchanged except for the patch of green paint, but Enos had a ruptured spleen, two broken kneecaps, and a squashed nose. He was fortunate that was the extent of it, as anybody knows who has tried to pick a fight with a bank.

Byrd and Avis were escorted by a trim, young secretary into the office of Llewellyn Cook, the bank treasurer. Mr. Cook shook hands with Byrd, bowed to Avis, and drew up two brown leather chairs for them beside his uncluttered mahogany desk. Cook was a tall, slim, middle-aged man with a shiny bald head, blue eyes, and an easy smile. He wore a flannel shirt, tweed jacket, khaki trousers, and boat shoes. His green necktie was secured with a clasp that bore the bank's logo. This was not at all what Byrd expected a banker to look like.

"Our appraiser has been out to the house, and he thinks the purchase price of $18,000 is about right," Cook said. "The bank can offer you a mortgage of $15,000 at 4.2% interest for twenty years with a $3,000 down payment. Does that seem reasonable to you folks?"

"That's fine with us," Byrd said. Three thousand dollars was all he had saved up to that time. Mr. Cook brought out the papers and was explaining the details of the mortgage, when a tall, rugged-looking old man strode into the banker's office, ignored Byrd and Avis, and went right up to lean his palms on Cook's desk. The old man had on muddy gum rubber boots, green woolen trousers, and a black and red plaid jacket. There was a faint but unmistakable odor of cow manure about his person.

"You're Mr. Cook?" he asked.

Cook allowed that he was.

"You probably don't remember it, but I was in here last fall when my money ran out, and I didn't have the bus fare to get back to my farm. You loaned me 85 cents, and I'm here to pay it back."

With that, he carefully placed a fifty-cent piece, a quarter, and a dime on the banker's desk, turned around, and walked out. Harry and Avis sat there stunned. Llewellyn Cook looked at them with a twinkle in his blue eyes. "I guess I'll have a piece of pie with my lunch today," he said.

After the papers were signed, Byrd again shook Cook's hand, and then he and Avis departed. As they drove away from the bank, he said, "Avis, I find it hard to believe that the old man, first of all, would go to a bank to borrow 85 cents; secondly, that the banker would lend it to him, and lastly, that he would come back six or seven months later to repay his debt. People here are certainly different from what I've been used to. In Boston the old guy would have been bounced out on his ear by a security guard."

"I felt a little bit like Alice in Wonderland," Avis said.

"I think we've come to the right place to live," said Harry.

The Huntress

It was the last poliomyelitis epidemic before the vaccine for that dread disease was developed. An entire floor of the hospital, namely Ward BX, was set aside for the care of desperately ill polio victims, many of them in primitive "iron lung" respirators like big green barrels with a bellows on one end to assist their breathing. Only the patient's head protruded from the other end of the barrel.

Dr. Harry Byrd, newly arrived in town, decided to take a shortcut through the polio ward. He knew it was a quarantine area, but he needed to get to the surgical suite in a hurry. Harry was tired, and it would be easier to go through it than around it. He pulled open the door of Ward BX and started down the corridor. Just then Nurse Kate McBreiarty came around the corner. She strongly resembled a full rigged sailing ship bearing down on him in her starched white uniform with the sleeves rolled up, white apron, white nurse's cap, white stockings and shoes. Her straight, gray hair was much shorter than the current style.

She was a very large woman, muscular, rather than obese. Byrd thought she was built like a lady wrestler, which would be a big advantage in hoisting around the polio patients and massaging and hot-packing their paralyzed limbs.

Kate bore down on Byrd and challenged him. Her words were like a shot fired across his bow.

"What are you doing on the isolation ward?"

"I'm Dr. Byrd, just on my way to the O.R.," he answered.

"I don't care if you're Dr. Louis Pasteur. Nobody comes on this floor who doesn't have business here. Go back around."

With that, she clamped a ham-like hand on his shoulder and steered him back out into the stairwell from whence he had come. Chastened, Byrd never tried that shortcut again.

In time he grew to appreciate Nurse Kate McBreiarty. She was always assigned to the toughest nursing problems and handled them well, with never a complaint. Injured drunks, wildly crazed with the D.T.'s (delirium tremens), were putty in her hands. Old ladies with fractured hips never developed bed sores when under her care because she hoisted them around to change their positions frequently and padded the pressure areas well. Her back rubs, or more accurately poundings, were stimulating to the circulation to say the least. She gave thorough bed baths and powdered all surfaces carefully. In fact, she was so liberal with the powder that Byrd sometimes thought her patients resembled powdered sugar crullers. Kate was tireless, cheerful, and devoted to her patients, constantly encouraging them and buoying up their spirits. They in turn responded and often recovered faster than expected. Kate was in her sixties and had never married. She lived with another large, tough single nurse, Dawn Brown. There were, of course, rumors about their association.

One day in the locker room Rodney Goshawk, the nose and throat surgeon, remarked to Byrd, "If you ask me, those old broads are a couple of perverted homoseckshuls."

"Rodney, I know what a homoseckshul is, but would you please explain to me what a perverted one is? Could that be heterosexual?" In Byrd's view their sexual preference made no difference because both women accomplished so much good in their life's work. As far as he was concerned, Kate's sexual preference, whether it was for men, women, or more likely neither, was none of his business.

In time Byrd's respect for Kate McBreiarty was reciprocated. She didn't seem to remember the episode on the polio ward. Kate liked the way he took care of his patients and the results he obtained. When she developed increasingly frequent episodes of abdominal pain that turned out to be due to gallstones, she asked Byrd to do the necessary surgery. As expected, Kate recovered quickly with little complaint about the unpleasant experience. She returned to the office for the follow-up visit.

"Are you progressing well, Kate?" Byrd asked.

"Oh, fine. I just tire a little easily."

"As you know, it'll be about six weeks before all your strength and energy return. You should stay out of work that long, and no lifting because it'll weaken your abdominal muscles," he said.

"I've been resting at camp. Dawn and I have a hunting camp out in Mariaville. Could you use some venison?"

"You go hunting?" he asked increduously.

"Oh sure, but it's no strain. There's a big apple tree right behind the camp. Dawn and I bring along a handful of Seconal sleeping capsules and stick one in each of the apples on the ground. The deer come around at night. They love apples, you know. Next morning we look out and there they are, fast asleep under the tree. We just open the window and KAPOW, we've got our deer." Then she added, "Don't tell anybody about it, though."

In those days sleeping pills were not closely monitored in the hospital as they are today. Nowadays, the nurses wouldn't be able to get away with that sort of pilfering. Kate brought in some nice venison steaks and chops at the time of her next visit. Byrd took them home, but he never did eat them because he was afraid he'd fall asleep right after dinner.

The Two-Dollar House Call

At the age of eighty Luther Crane continued an active general practice of medicine with emphasis on obstetrics. He was always available, day or night, including holidays and weekends. When one of his maternity patients in active labor entered the hospital, he stayed with her constantly until she had given birth, and he was satisfied that all was well with both mother and child. In his younger years he did a considerable volume of surgery— always carefully, efficiently, and with meticulous technique. His patients with more complex operative problems were referred by him to more highly qualified surgical specialists, but he continued to visit and encourage those patients through the recovery period and beyond. They remained his patients.

Luther Crane's office was in a big, yellow house where he lived at the top of a hill on the edge of town. He was a bachelor, and his spinster sister kept house for him. He said he had never needed a wife because he was married to his profession. He loved his patients and they, in return, loved him. When new, young physicians settled in the community, he helped train and advise them, as long as he considered them properly qualified and motivated. He shunned any young doctor who he suspected was primarily selfishly interested in the accumulation of wealth at the expense of sick people and who failed to treat patients with care and respect.

One evening young Doctor Byrd was making his evening rounds to check on postoperative patients, and to examine and instruct those who were preoperative. As he walked along the corridor on the surgical floor of the hospital, he met Doctor Luther Crane who was strolling in the opposite direction. The elderly physician was a small man, slight of build, with gray hair and mustache. Wire-rimmed, round bifocal spectacles were perched on his nose. He was dressed in pajamas, slippers, and a long, brown, heavy bathrobe with braided rope belt and piping. As usual he appeared relaxed and was smiling.

"I'm sorry to see you here, Dr. Crane," Byrd said.

Crane peered over the top of his spectacles at the young man. "Why should you be sorry? I've been coming here every day for the last fifty years," he said.

"Yes, but not as a patient," Byrd said.

"It's good for a man to see life from another perspective once in awhile. I've never been sick in my life before, but lately my gallbladder has been acting up. It's full of rocks. My old friend George Eagleton will be taking it out in the morning."

Eagleton was an old-time surgeon of Crane's generation who was considered by those who knew him as the fastest man in the East. He had to be fast in his earlier years because he often went out into the countryside with his nurse etherizer to do operations. On the patient's kitchen table Eagleton would perform an appendectomy, a tonsillectomy, drainage of abscessed ears, and other surgical procedures. Byrd's generation of surgeons, with the advantage of refined anesthesia techniques, was taught to emphasize safety and accuracy rather than speed. Home surgery was no longer acceptable. That very morning Byrd had assisted Eagleton at a Caesarean section. While they scrubbed up at the sink outside the operating room, Eagleton had a lit cigarette dangling from his mouth. When it burned down to a short stubb, the nurse came over, snuffed it out, and pulled up the surgeon's mask over his face. Eagleton went into the operating room. By the time Byrd had finished scrubbing and the nurse had gowned and gloved him, the old man had prepared the patient's skin with antiseptic solution, draped the abdomen, and made a single sweep of the scalpel through skin, fat, muscle, and peritoneum. As Byrd bellied up to the table, there was another sweep of the scalpel through the uterus. Out popped a healthy pink infant without a scratch on him and bawling in protest at being rudely snatched from his cozy, warm, and watery home in the womb. Eagleton had foresightedly tilted the table toward the side of his assistant standing across from him, so that the flood of blood and amniotic fluid ran all over Byrd's front and not his own. After the umbilical cord had been cut and the placenta removed, the healthy baby was passed off the table into a blanket held by the attending pediatrician. The two surgeons suctioned and sponged up the field. The incisions in the uterus and abdominal wall were sutured closed, and the dressings were applied. In the locker room Byrd looked at the clock and shook his head in disbelief. The entire operation had taken only twenty minutes!

"Well, I'm sure you'll do well tomorrow," Byrd said to Luther Crane. "You've stayed in great shape."

"Yes, I've always exercised regularly, and I've never been a big eater. As you well know, fat is the enemy of the surgeon."

"That's a handsome bathrobe you're wearing," Byrd said.

"Had it for years. You can't buy them like this anymore. My pajamas are brand new, though. Did you ever notice when men come in to the hospital, they always wear new pajamas, unless they come in for an emergency? I suppose that's because the old ones are worn out and unpresentable, or else they don't wear any at home. Women, on the other hand, always come in with their hair freshly coiffed. The last thing they do before being admitted to the hospital is visit the 'New You Beauty Salon' or some other hairdressing establishment."

"I hadn't thought about that, but it is true, now that you mention it," Byrd said. "Do you plan to go back to full time practice after the operation?"

"Of course! I plan to stay out about six weeks. As you know, obstetrics is my first love. The breeders are poor, and often I don't get paid, but it's a great satisfaction to know that the life you help come into the world goes on for three quarters of a century on average. When you operate on someone in their sixties to eighties, a few years may be added to that person's life, but most of that life has already gone by. There is satisfaction for you there, but it's not as great as it is in obstetrics. I've arranged with the obstetricians to take care of my maternity cases until I get back. My other patients can get along without me for awhile. If they get into difficulties, they can call on someone else to tide them over."

Early the next morning Luther Crane underwent removal of his gallbladder, and also removal of two stones that had worked their way down from the gallbladder into his bile duct. Byrd was gratified to learn that the old gentleman did well, had no complications, and went home to convalesce.

Several weeks later a call came to Byrd's office from Mrs. Mordecai Mudgett.

"What's the problem, Mrs. Mudgett?" he asked.

"Mordecai has diabetes. Dr. Luther Crane taught him how to take care of it. He follows the diet, tests his urine, and I give him the insulin shots," she said.

"So that's not a problem, is it?" he asked.

"I'm coming to that. For the last three days his foot hurts. It's all swollen and red. I told him not to pare that corn on the bottom behind his big toe, but he's so contrary that he just had to go ahead and do it. Now he's got himself into a mess."

"Can you bring him to my office this afternoon?"

"I don't see how I can. We don't have a car, and I don't drive, anyway. He can't step on it because it hurts, so there's no way I can get him out to a taxicab. Doctor Crane always comes out to the house when we need him."

"All right. I'll be there this evening after office hours. Where do you live?"

"We're up on the hill behind the Unitarian Church, 30 Cedar Street."

Byrd went up the granite steps of the Mudgett home at 6 pm. It was an old frame house set close to the sidewalk and wedged between two other old houses along the street. Mrs. Mudgett answered the doorbell and ushered him in. She was a thin, gray haired lady and was wearing a print dress. The house was neat, clean, and sparsely furnished. There was linoleum on the floor and no rugs. Framed pictures of the city in the old days hung on the walls. The patient was sitting in a wing back chair, fiddling with the dial of a large Philco radio on the pine table beside him. The infected foot was immersed in a pan of water on the floor. Doctor Byrd pulled up a chair and sat next to Mr. Mudgett.

"Do you folks live here alone in this big house?" he asked.

"No, we take in roomers," Mordecai said. "They're all old men like me, but widowed or divorced. Helps Minnie and me a bit with our bills and taxes. My social security payments don't go far these days."

"What kind of work did you do before you retired?" Byrd asked.

"I was a woodsman and guide. Our roomers mostly worked in the woods, too. They were a wild bunch in their younger days, but now the sap's run out of them, and they're just waiting for the grim reaper like we are."

"Is your diabetes under control?"

"It is now. The urine sugar tests are green, but I had to up the insulin some the past two days. It was testing orange."

24

"That's because of the infection. Let me just get a look at that foot."

Mordecai lifted his dripping foot out of the pan of water, and his wife dried it gently with a towel. There was redness and swelling of the foot, and a couple of red lines extended up toward the ankle. Byrd felt for the pulses on top of the foot and behind the inner part of the ankle bone. He noted with relief that the pulses were present, although weak. Arteriosclerosis had impaired but not shut down the blood flow to the old man's foot, so that ischemic gangrene was not too much of a threat. There were some swollen lymph glands in the groin, indicating the body's attempt to block spread of the infection above the lower limb. A thermometer placed under Mordecai's tongue indicated that there was no fever.

Byrd prescribed an antibiotic and gave the couple the name of a pharmacy that would deliver it. He instructed Mordecai to lie on the couch with his foot elevated rather than sit with it dangling down. Elevation would help reduce the swelling. Also, he advised continuation of the soaks, or warm wet packs, but to use tepid rather than hot water which increases tissue metabolism in the foot. "With impaired circulation this might be damaging to the tissues because the blood supply was exceeded by the demand for it," Bryd explained.

"How much do we owe you, Doctor?" Mrs. Mudgett asked, as Bryd rose to leave.

"I'll charge you the same as Dr. Crane does," he answered. She opened her purse and peeled off two one dollar bills from a modest wad of greenbacks.

"Thank you for coming, Doctor," she said.

"You're quite welcome, and I believe Dr. Crane will be back in action in a few days. Please let him know how things are progressing. If you need me before that, just give a call. I'll be around."

Two weeks later, Harry Byrd met Luther Crane again in the hospital corridor. This time the old gentleman was nattily attired in a brown, herringbone tweed jacket and charcoal gray flannel slacks. His maroon necktie had miniature flying ducks printed all over it and a hardly noticeable soup stain. He was making his rounds to visit his hospitalized patients.

"Glad to see you back, Dr. Crane," Byrd said.

"Never felt better in my life," Crane said, peering over the top of his spectacles at the young surgeon. "Thanks for seeing my friend Mordecai Mudgett while I was laid up. He's fine now. And oh, by the way, you got cheated."

"What?"

"Yes, it's two dollars for an office visit. I always charge three for a house call."

Ten years later, Luther Crane died peacefully at the age of ninety, quite content that he had accomplished his goals in life. But there was more. He bequeathed his entire estate to the hospital where he had cared for the sick for so many years. The value of the estate was half a million dollars. It was stipulated in the will that the income from the estate be used for the support of needy patients.

Harry Byrd and his wife were discussing the bequest one morning at breakfast. "How do you suppose, Avis, that Luther Crane ever accumulated an estate that large on two dollar office calls and delivering babies? Half of his patients couldn't afford to pay him, and he took care of them the same way as the ones who did pay. I have an idea that Luther made some wise investments, especially in the early days when taxes were low. He probably figured that some day everyone would own an automobile and have a telephone in the house, so he bought stock in companies like Ford Motors and AT&T. He may have seemed old fashioned, but he read a lot and kept up to date on world developments. It wouldn't surprise me if he had bought stocks like I.B.M. and Xerox when they were in their infancy."

"Well, for one thing," Avis said, "he never spent any money. He lived frugally and never went anywhere that I know of. His avocation was the same as his vocation. There was never a wife to support and children to raise."

"I used to think that each one of our children was worth a million dollars. Now that we've raised them to be honest citizens, and they've all completed their education, I still think that, but I also think that each of them cost a million dollars, or close to it," Harry said. "I'm not in any way advocating celibacy or the complete lack of diversion from the practice of medicine. Luther Crane went to extremes in his devotion to his patients. But any young doctor coming along could learn an awful lot about life from that man. I know I did. Most people at the end of their lives leave children as their legacy. Some leave creative works like art, music, and literature. Luther Crane's legacy is the continuing care of the patients he lived for."

27

The Cover Up

The single Latin word inscribed on the emblem of his alma mater - Veritas - often came to the mind of Harry Byrd. He regarded the search for truth as a very serious matter. Truth and honesty were virtues to be cherished. He was deeply impressed during surgical residency training when the professor, who was a world-famed authority in surgery of the pancreas, stood up at a mortality meeting where patient deaths are analyzed in detail and calmly stated in front of his students and fellow teachers that the death of a man whose pancreas he had recently removed was due to a technical error made by himself. The professor was teaching by example. Never after that day was Byrd ashamed or reluctant to admit his own errors. He listened with scorn to those prima donna surgeons who sometimes went to elaborate lengths to disguise or explain away the untoward results caused by their errors of omission or commission, often blaming their assistants, faulty instruments, nursing care, and sometimes even the patients themselves.

That is not to say, however, that Byrd was guiltless, as exemplified by the case of a certain student nurse. Early one evening in the first year of his surgical practice, Byrd was called by Charley Robbins, the young internist who was assigned to look after the health of the young women in the hospital's school of nursing.

"Would you be willing to see a student nurse I've just admitted to the hospital with abdominal pain, possibly appendicitis?" Charley asked.

"Be right up. Where is she?"

"Ward S. I'll be waiting here."

Byrd found Robbins sitting in the nurse's station looking worried.

"The girl's name is Phoebe Danforth. She's twenty years old and never been sick in her life. I won't tell you my findings until after you've evaluated the situation. Might prejudice you. The lab studies should be back soon."

Byrd was accompanied by Sylvia Lang, the middle-aged, widowed nurse in charge of the ward during the evening shift. She opened the door of the patient's room and said, "Here's Dr. Byrd."

There was an absolutely beautiful, slim, young woman lying quietly in the austere white hospital bed. Her long, black, glossy hair was spread out over the pillow, and she held the sheet up tightly to her chin, as she looked at Byrd apprehensively. Her green eyes were unusually shiny, he noted. He had never read it anywhere in a book but had often observed that people with inflammation going on in the abdomen have abnormally shiny eyes.

"Hello, Phoebe. Where's your home?" he asked.

"Wytopitlock, up north in Aroostook County. You've probably never heard of it," she said.

"Oh, yes. I took care of a woodsman from up there last winter. He had frostbitten feet, and we had to amputate three of his toes."

"Everybody knows everybody else up home," she said. "What's his name?"

"Harold Morgan."

"Harold used to work for my father," she said.

"What kind of work does your dad do?"

"He runs a sawmill."

"How did you happen to go into nursing?"

"I've always wanted to be a nurse. It just makes me happy to see sick people get well, especially if I've been part of their getting well."

"When do you graduate?"

"Next June. I'm a senior."

"Do you have a steady boyfriend?"

"I did but we broke up a while back. He's from up home and sort of, you might say, too provincial. Lately, I've gone out a few times with a fighter pilot from the Air Force base. He's from California originally, but he's been all over the world. I love to just listen to his stories. They're wonderful and exciting."

Byrd figured that the ice had been broken at least a little bit with Phoebe, so he got down to the problem at hand. "Tell me about this pain," he said.

"Well, it started this morning down here on the right side. It got steadily worse all day and spread over to the left. I walk all bent over. It feels better if I lie still."

"Does it hurt when you cough?"

"I don't have a cough." She gave a little cough, and her face contorted with obvious pain.

"Any nausea or vomiting?"

"No, but I haven't felt like eating anything all day."

"Are your bowels all right?"

"Fine. I went this morning, same as every day."

"Any urinary symptoms?"

"No, but I had some burning and frequency for a few days last week."

"How about the periods?"

"Perfectly regular, as usual."

"Any discharge?"

"Some. Just since my last period ten days ago. It's sort of off-white."

Byrd then examined Phoebe, starting at the head and neck, then worked down. Everything was quite normal until he reached the abdomen. There was tenderness with involuntary muscle spasm in the lower abdomen on the right, less pronounced on the left. Sudden release of manual pressure on both sides produced the same pain as the previous cough, caused by friction of the lining surfaces inside the abdomen against each other and indicative of inflammatory changes. Byrd always had the rather naive idea that a pelvic examination on young, unmarried female should be avoided. In this instance, however, it was obviously an important part of the examination. The nurse carefully draped the patient with a sheet over her abdomen and flexed thighs to protect her modesty. The examining finger was easily passed into the pelvis without a hymenal barrier being encountered. There was a little yellowish discharge in the mouth of the cervix of the uterus, and digital pressure on the cervix produced what is known as the "chandelier sign." That is to say, when there is inflammation in the pelvis, motion of the uterus causes such pain that the patient goes up toward the ceiling, and if there happens to be a chandelier there, swings from it. The uterus was normal size, and the fallopian tubes on each side of it were very tender.

"I'm sorry that hurt you, Phoebe, but it's necessary to figure out what's wrong."

Byrd rejoined Robbins back at the nursing station.

"The lab reports came in," Robbins said. "No anemia, white blood cell count is up, and so is the sedimentation rate. The quickie pregnancy test is negative. A few pus cells in the urine. What do you think?"

"I don't believe it's appendicitis. Looks like gonorrhea that has gone up through the uterus and tubes to produce pelvic inflammation."

"That's what I think, too. I purposely didn't do a smear test yet on that discharge to look for gonorrhea organisms. Now, I also think that since we are both young guys starting out, and this is a nursing student, it might be best to get confirmation from a greybeard."

Robbins telephoned Artemus Bulfinch, the gynecologist who was a big, gruff, but kindly teddy bear of a man, in his early sixties. Artemus was at a dinner party but agreed to come right over when he was told the situation. He went directly to the patient's room, and the nurse again placed the drape sheet over Phoebe. The two young doctors watched.

"Oh, not again," groaned Phoebe.

Artemus grabbed the sheet, threw it on the floor in the corner, and mumbled, "That's like taking a bath with your socks on."

He quickly examined the girl's abdomen and pelvis, then beckoned the two young doctors out into the corridor.

"What is your opinion, Dr. Bulfinch?" Robbins asked.

"Couldn't be anything but the clap," Bulfinch said, and then he walked off to the elevator. "Missed the shrimp cocktail, but if I hurry, they'll just be serving the roast beef."

"Thanks for your help," Byrd said.

"When the director of student nurses finds out about this, she'll surely throw Phoebe out of the program. That's an awful price to pay for a roll in the hay," Robbins said.

"Maybe you should take her appendix out anyway, give her the right antibiotic, and she'll be cured."

"You know I can't do that, Charley," Byrd said, "but we can't let this kid's future be ruined." He knew the strict, old spinster director would drop the girl from the training program if she knew about this. In fact, she once nearly fired the student who was babysitting for the Byrd children and got back to the dormitory ten minutes after the 11:00 p.m. curfew, even though Byrd testified that it was his fault, not the student's. What the hell was she supposed to do, leave the children stranded?

"You notice, Charley, that Dr. Bulfinch didn't write anything in the patient's chart. Do you suppose he was just interested in getting back for the roast beef, or was that a hint to us? Now listen, there were some pus cells in the urine, even though not many, and, no doubt, just a contamination from the other problem when she urinated. Let's call this a urinary tract infection for the record and treat her with the right antibiotic for the other problem."

Charley's worried face broke into a broad smile. "That's it, Harry. Meanwhile, I'll get the name of that flyboy, call up Tony Plover, the flight surgeon out at the base, and have that California guy treated before he infects half of the County."

"They say that California is ten years ahead of Maine as far as progress goes, but not everything they export to us is beneficial," Byrd said.

They looked across the station at Sylvia Lang who was carefully engrossed in another patient's chart and trying not to overhear them. They knew she had raised a couple of daughters alone after the death of her husband. She was smiling and nodding her head slightly. Without a doubt, she agreed with the plan. Benjamin Franklin once said that three can keep a secret if two are dead. Old Ben was wrong this time. Phoebe rapidly regained her health and graduated with her nursing school class.

About a year later, Harry Byrd was reading the morning paper at breakfast. It was a Saturday, the day the newspaper devoted a page to the recent weddings, engagements, and a few fifty year marriages. His wife Avis always read that page carefully, although Harry usually skipped right over it. A familiar face caught his eye. The beautiful bride smiling at him from the photograph was Phoebe Danforth. Beneath the picture was the usual, detailed description of the wedding. Byrd was please to note that the groom was a recent graduate of the venerable

Union Theological Seminary in Albany, New York. He silently wished the handsome, young couple a long and happy life together. And he hoped that the Veritas emblem wasn't too tarnished.

My Wife's Second Husband

Harry Byrd looked across his cluttered desk at an impressive, elderly couple holding hands and sitting beside each other in red leather chairs. Ira Hardy looked much younger than his seventy-two years. He was of medium height, lean, and trim, although pale. His face was unwrinkled except for crow's feet at the corners of his eyes, suggesting a man of good humor who smiled often. Most of his hair was gone except for a gray lock in the middle of the scalp on top, which brought to mind a kewpie doll. He had a habit of arching his eyebrows and wrinkling his forehead briefly, which gave him a surprised look and brought the lock of hair on top forward, then backward. His wife, Amy, must have been a stunning beauty in her youth and in her later years was still a lovely woman. They appeared relaxed in spite of knowing that Ira had a serious problem. His family doctor had found that Ira had anemia of the type due to chronic occult blood loss. Studies disclosed the source to be in the large intestine. There was a cauliflower-like growth, most likely malignant.

"How long have you folks been married?" Byrd asked.

"Fifty-two years," Ira said. "Amy was only seventeen at the time, and they all said I was robbing the cradle, but it seems to have worked out all right." He turned to his wife, and they smiled at each other, eyes twinkling.

"Half a century proves that pretty well," Byrd replied. "Nowadays people seem to shed spouses like they would an old suit of clothes, then go out to get a new one."

"We raised four children together. They're all good, honest citizens and out on their own now," Ira said.

"Yes, and we have nine grandchildren," Amy added.

"What kind of work did you do over the years, Mr. Hardy?" Byrd asked.

"Worked for the hydroelectric company. I was a lineman for years. When I got older, they were afraid I'd fall off a pole or something, so they moved me into the shop until I retired. Now, we live up here at our camp on Whetstone Pond in the summer. I can catch me a nice fat trout right from my front dooryard. In the winter we go to Zephyrhills down in Florida."

"Quite a few Mainers go there, don't they?" Byrd said.

"Most everybody lives in one of the trailer parks down there, but where we stay, they're not all on top of one another. It's well-landscaped. In fact, there's a grapefruit tree right alongside the trailer. We eat off it all winter, even get cankers in the mouth from eating too many, if we're not careful. Why they call that place Zephyrhills, I'll never know, unless it's to attract people from the North. There are plenty of zephyrs all right, but the hills seem about twenty feet high at the most. When we first drove down there, we noticed that the whole State of Florida is flat as a pancake. One time, off in the distance, we saw a hill, and my heart jumped at the sight, but when we got closer, it turned out to be a giant refuse dump that looked like a big cake with alternating layers of sand and trash. An old, yellow bulldozer was pushing stuff up the hill as a flock of seagulls flew around the top looking for goodies. Probably a thousand years from now, the archeologists will go digging around in those dumps to learn about our civilization, just like they do now in the old Indian shell heaps along the Maine coast."

"Now, tell me what you've had for illnesses in the past, Mr. Hardy," Byrd said.

"Nuthin'. Never hardly been sick a day in my life except for maybe a cold every once in a while, and I did mash my thumb once. See, it's still kind of flat on the end," as he held up the spoon-shaped member.

"How did you notice this trouble that you have now?"

"Well, I couldn't hardly get my chores done around camp without being all pooped out. Just walking down to the mailbox made me feel all used up."

"And he began to look awfully peaked around the gills," Amy added, "so I made him go to see my doctor."

"Well, as Dr. Godwit explained to you, the trouble is in the lower part of your intestines." Byrd drew a diagram of the abdomen with the intestine arranged within it. "It's a growth here on the right side next to the appendix, and it just keeps leaking blood in such small amounts that you can't even see it, but in time it drains your blood way down. We need to remove this section of the bowel and connect the ends back together again. There's a good chance that will cure the problem." He went on to explain in detail what Ira could expect about the planned operation and convalescent period.

"I'm not worried, even if worst comes to worst," Ira said. "You know, Doctor, I believe in reincarnation. In my next life I'd like to come back as my wife's second husband." His eyebrows went up, and his scalp moved forward, then back.

Byrd looked at Amy who was smiling tolerantly at her husband's foolishness. "I guess, Mrs. Hardy, that's about the highest compliment a man could give a woman," he said.

She nodded in agreement and laughed. Ira Hardy was admitted to the hospital, and after several pints of blood replacement transfusion, as well as preparation of the bowel with cleansing and antibiotics, the right half of his large intestine was removed. The growth was malignant, but fortunately, it was relatively superficial and appeared not to have spread. Ira recovered rapidly after the operation with few complaints and hardly ever losing his smile. Amy was in constant attendance, reading or knitting in a chair near the window overlooking the river and the green hills beyond. She expressed appreciation for Ira's caring nurses who "seemed almost like family" and brought them a large box of Russell Stover chocolates. Byrd gave the couple a thorough, encouraging report and advised Ira to return periodically for follow-up examinations and tests for the next thirty years. He didn't really expect that either he or his patient would live that long, but the implication was that the problem was cured, and this never failed to reassure the patient, even though it produced a smile.

The Hardys came in for the scheduled office visit after their return from Florida during the following spring. "What kind of winter did you have?" Byrd asked, observing that they both looked quite well.

"We had a frost in January that froze our grapefruit and killed the tree," Ira said, "and it was right after that when I had the heart attack."

"Tell me about that."

"The tree?"

"No, the heart attack."

"Well, I was digging in the garden, and this wicked pressure came in the front of my chest, like a horse was sitting on it. Amy drove me to the hospital, and they took a cardiogram. The doctor gave me morphine and oxygen. Then, I was in the intensive care unit on a monitor for a few days. After that, they transferred me to a room, and the next day the funniest thing happened."

"What was that?" Byrd asked.

"Well, I was sitting on the edge of the bed, and Amy was over by the window reading when all of a sudden I checked out." Ira's eyebrows went up, and his scalp came forward, then back.

"What!"

"Yes, he just keeled over backwards on the bed," Amy said. "Then this big fat nurse came running in with a plywood plank, shoved it under him, jumped up on top, pounded him on the chest, then began pushing on him and blowing air down his throat. It wasn't more than a couple of minutes before a whole troop of people came in with the crash cart, and that's when he woke up."

"First thing I remember," Ira said, "was this big nurse with her white dress hiked up practically to her hips, straddling me and pushing on my chest. She was red in the face, and her nurse's cap was falling off sideways. She started to hold my nose and blow air in my mouth. So I said, 'Does this mean we're engaged?'"

"How did she respond to that?" Byrd asked.

"She said, 'You old bastard, you'll never die!'"

Byrd glanced over at Amy, who was smiling as usual and nodding to confirm her husband's description of the wild scene.

"Isn't he awful," she said.

"Well, I didn't have anymore trouble after that, never a twinge of pain, and I'm fine now, four months later." His eyebrows went up again.

Byrd examined his patient and arranged for some studies which all turned out well. After that they met again every year. There was no evidence of recurrent cancer, and there were no further heart problems. Then one summer morning at breakfast, Byrd was saddened to read his friend Ira's obituary in the daily newspaper. After completing the morning's surgery he went to the medical floor at the hospital where Lisa Hardy, Ira's daughter-in-law, worked as a nurse.

"What happened?" he asked Lisa, who looked sad.

"Well, Gramps took his grandson, Billy, fishing Saturday. After dinner the two of them were in the sitting room watching "Murder She Wrote". When the program was over, Billy got up to switch off the TV. Gramps was just sitting there in the armchair, smiling, but he didn't answer when Billy spoke to him. That was it. He was gone."

"Nice and easy for him," Byrd said, "but what about Amy?"

"She's taking it well," Lisa said. "Keeps talking about all those good years they had together, but of course, it's hard on her."

"Yes, I understand," Byrd said. "Is she still smiling?"

"You know it!"

Amy never did have a second husband. She joined Ira a few years later, peacefully.

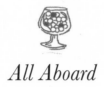

All Aboard

Some years back there was a tough, old Piscataquis County physician, named George Fisher. His patients were scattered over a large, thinly populated area of lakes and forests. It didn't matter to him that many of them couldn't and didn't pay his modest bills because they were almost all hard-working, honest people who could make it all right financially when they were well, but when they were sick or injured, they quickly became broke. In those days few people had private health insurance, and government programs such as Medicaid and Medicare hadn't even been thought of yet. The small local hospital had very limited facilities, so Fisher referred his complicated problems to the hospital in Bangor, thirty-five miles to the south. Among others, Harry Byrd took care of Fisher's surgical problems, and he too treated the patients who couldn't pay their medical bills the same way as those who could, namely as friends who needed his help. This was not lost on George Fisher who paid Byrd the ultimate compliment—he invited him to go fishing at his camp on a remote lake, or as he put it, "Come on up and wet a line with me."

So one bright spring morning after the ice had gone out of the lakes, Byrd drove up to Piscataquis County and met with Fisher. Together they went over dirt roads that were hard packed by lumber trucks and arrived at Fisher's camp on the shore of a lake that sparkled like a jewel in the sunshine. The lake was surrounded by fragrant evergreen woods, and Boarstone Mountain rose in the background. It was a scene of isolated and unmarred, primitive beauty except for one thing, a pair of glistening steel rails on a gravel roadbed passing between the cabin and the shore of the lake.

The two men crossed over the rails, got into an old flat-bottomed rowboat on the shore with their fishing gear, stowed their lunch under a thwart in a Coleman cooler, then shoved off onto the lake. Fisher was an expert fly fisherman, and Byrd managed to cast his fly without fouling his companion's lines or worse, hooking or snagging him with a hook. He watched Fisher flick the line in the air behind him in a graceful arc, then cast it far out forward onto the water's smooth surface, and reel the fly back slowly toward the boat.

"Look here, Harry," he said, watching the flailing action of his inexperienced friend's casting. "Don't try to beat the fish to death like that. You're supposed to be luring him to the hook. The secret is all in the wrist motion, like this."

Under George's expert tutelage Byrd soon had a strike. The trout broke the surface of the water, and the reel whirred as the fish dove to rid itself of the hook. "Keep your tip up," said Fisher, as the rod arched downward, "and don't let the line go slack. Keep reeling it in steady." Gradually, the trout was brought close to the boat, and Fisher netted it.

During the course of the day they caught the legal limit of ten to twelve-inch fat trout, most of them hooked by Fisher. They talked of many things while the boat drifted in the soft breeze.

"Tell me about that railroad track, George," Byrd said. "It seems sort of strange out here in the middle of nowhere."

Fisher explained in his usual roundabout fashion. "If you look at the map of the forty-eight contiguous states, you see three obvious projections. First, there's Texas, extending down into Mexico like the keel of a sailboat. Then, there's Florida, dangling down like a penis from the nether regions of the nation. It's a regular phallic symbol in more ways than one. Lastly, there's Maine, sticking into Canada's underside like a big thumb.

"What's all that got to do with the railroad?" Byrd asked.

"I'm coming to that. This thumb, which is Maine, poses some problems. You notice all the paved roads in northern Maine, what there are of them, run north and south. An east to west highway across northern Maine would open it up for development and probably ruin it. As of now, only the Canadian Pacific Railroad traverses the State across the midsection, east and west. Otherwise, freight and passenger trains traveling between the Maritime Provinces and Quebec, thence to western Canada, would have to travel hundreds of miles out of their direct route, up one side and down the other of the big old thumb. Of course, each time a train crosses the State, it has to go over the border through Customs at McAdam, New Brunswick and Vanceboro, Maine in the east and Lowelltown, Maine and Megantic, Quebec in the west because it travels through a foreign country. What you're looking at right in front of my fishing camp in the middle of all this natural beauty is the main rail line between Halifax, Nova Scotia on Canada's east coast and Vancouver, British Columbia on the west coast. I've taken that train trip across Canada, and some places along the line out west are even more beautiful than this, especially in the Canadian Rockies."

In the late afternoon the men rowed back to camp, cleaned their fish at the water's edge, and packed them on ice in the cooler. Fisher produced a bottle of Canadian whiskey from the cabin and poured them each half a tumblerful. They sat there on the porch, feet up on the railing, chairs tilted back, hats tilted forward, just looking out at the shining lake through narrowed eyelids, enjoying the late afternoon coolness and the sweet smell of the forest.

The silence was broken by the distant piercing wail of a whistle coming from the east. "That'll be the crack flyer coming through," Fisher said. "They carry freight from the ports of Halifax and St. John right across to the west coast of Canada. Proud of their speed, they are, going across."

Soon they could hear the harsh sound of diesel engines gradually becoming louder, and then two giant locomotives, in tandem, with freight cars behind, came into view. They were going very slowly, which surprised Byrd since this was the speedy transcontinental flyer. The engines screeched to a stop right in front of the camp, blocking the view. The diesels rumbled impatiently, and the fumes of their exhaust polluted the pure air. The entire crew of the train climbed down and came up on Fisher's porch, smiling broadly. He greeted them, introduced each by name to Harry, and they shook hands all around. The crew members were a tough, rugged, jovial bunch. They all had a drink, and Byrd thought to himself that Fisher must, of course, have produced some iced tea from within the cabin. Then off they went, heading for the Onawa trestle, Bodfish Valley, Greenville Junction, and the Canadian border. The freight cars clicked over the rails as they passed in a seemingly endless parade, then finally the caboose disappeared to the west. Byrd envisioned the board of directors of the railroad sitting in their plush offices in Montreal or wherever they were, and he wondered what their reaction would be if they had been aware of this unscheduled wilderness stop for refreshment.

"They'll make up the time easily," Fisher said, reading Byrd's thoughts.

"How do you know all those men, George?"

"There is a big railroad facility at Brownville Junction, halfway across the State and right in my practice area. I've taken care of the railroad men and their families for years. Engineers, firemen, conductors, trackmen, gandy dancers, mechanics, you name it. They all live around here to maintain and repair the trains, tracks, and roadbed. In fact, the first time I met those boys was when I held them upside down by the heels and whacked their bottoms to introduce them to the world."

By this time the sun was low on the horizon in an orange sky, layered with flat purple clouds. Fisher divided the trout equally, and the two men left the fishing camp.

Harry Byrd would fondly remember that day for the rest of his life.

The Weir Man

Benjamin Caldwell was a gentle giant of a man, sort of a cross between John Wayne and Merlin Olson. He had lived all his life just off the Maine coast on an island connected by a long arching bridge. He loved his island and the sea where he earned his livelihood. The green island was blanketed with symmetrical fir trees and jagged, irregular, tall pines where eagles nested. Granite cliffs rose above the surf on the seaward side with several snug harbors and pebble beaches on the leeward side of the island. Gulls, wheeling and screaming for a handout of discarded fish, drifted on the air currents or followed in the wake of fishing boats. The dense fog that often rolled in to enshroud the island for prolonged periods and the bitter winter with its storms that raged in from the Atlantic didn't bother Caldwell nor reduce his appreciation of the beauty that surrounded him.

In his youth he had worked as crewman on a trawler. Then he built his own weir in the shallow water of a cove on the island. Hundreds of years earlier, the English settlers had learned and refined the method of weir fishing, developed by the Indians who called themselves "the People of the Dawn." The English gave the tribes less romantic names, according to the bodies of water nearby, such as Penobscot or Passamaquoddy. Benjamin felled young trees in the forest, fashioned them into poles and drove them into the muddy bottom of the cove with a pile driver to form a circle with an open gap facing the shore. He strung nets on these poles around the circumference, extending upward from the floor of the cove where they were weighted securely with rocks to a level above the high tide mark. The tides were eighteen feet or more on this part of the coast so the poles had to be long and sturdy. In the center of the gap he placed a straight row of poles and netting extending radially outward from the circle to form a "leader" into the enclosure. The whole thing was like an electronic Pacman game except that it stayed in one place with its mouth open instead of traveling around gobbling things up.

Every year in the summer, usually once, sometimes twice, and one year not at all, great schools of young herring, sometimes pursued by larger predatory fish, came in from the bay to feed on plankton in the relatively warm shallow water. In the space of a few hours great numbers of the herring would suddenly come into the weir along the leader, fill it to capacity, and swim around in circles. Trapped by the nets, the fish were unable to figure the way back out through the entrance. The weir man would observe the boiling turmoil on the surface of the water from the fish thrashing inside the weir. Then, he would call in his friend who owned a sardine carrier. Soon, the sixty-foot, diesel-powered, wooden boat would heave to at the weir. The crew would lower a big vacuum pipe on a boom into the shimmering mass of fish churning the water and pump them into the boat's hold. First, a layer of fish was deposited in the hold. Then the crew emptied bags of salt on top of them, followed by another layer of fish, alternating that way until the hold was filled, and the boat lay low in the water. The loaded sardine carrier would chug off to the dockside sardine cannery. There the fish were unloaded into hogsheads, each weighing half a ton when full. During processing, the fish were passed along on a conveyer belt in front of women workers who, without ever losing a finger, scissored off the heads and tails and packed them side by side like sardines, which they were, into flat cans with soya oil. Sometimes, mustard or Louisiana hot sauce was added to tickle the palate. Then, the cans of sardines were steam-cooked and ready for market. The heads and tails were sold to the lobstermen as bait for their traps. Piles of residual, shining scales went to the pearl essence plant to be processed into paint ingredients and costume jewelry among other things. Nothing was wasted except the fish smell, which was not exactly marketable. In one day Benjamin Caldwell's weir could yield 300 to 500 hogsheads of sardines, each worth $85 more or less. Forty-thousand dollars in one day wasn't too bad a return on his initial investment in nets, poles, and the pile driver. Of course, Ben had to check the weir regularly, repair holes in the nets, and replace poles that were damaged by storms. Not infrequently, harbor seals swam into the weir. Since they were much bigger and smarter than herring, the seals easily figured a way out. Their favorite tactic was to grab a hold on the twine, spin around a few times, and rip a hole right through it.

Benjamin Caldwell had a severe aversion to hospitals and doctors, and that was quite understandable in view of his past experience. He had been born with a serious physical deformity. When he was a small boy of eight years, he had been sent to a world famous-teaching hospital in Boston where renowned surgeons corrected the deformity in a prolonged and intricate operation. The surgeons were quite proud of their accomplishment and presented their case to an audience of visiting doctors, resident surgeons, and medical students in a big amphitheater at the hospital. Benjamin was wheeled in and had to lie there, completely exposed, with hundreds of dispassionate eyes staring down at the boy while his surgeon displayed the marvelous achievement and described the advanced surgical technique he had developed. What they all failed to realize was that the shy island boy, who was at home with the sea and fog, the wind, the cliffs, and the evergreen trees of his island, was completely terrorized by this experience that made him feel like some kind of freak of nature. And of course, he was not. While treating his body, the doctors overlooked something equally important, namely his mind. Their goal was to achieve a long, healthy life for their patient, but instead, as it turned out, they unwittingly doomed him to a premature death. Young Benjamin vowed to himself that he would sooner die than to go near another hospital.

Caldwell grew up to be taller, stronger, and more handsome than the other island boys. He fell in love with and married Rachel Wilson to whom he was devoted for life, as she was to him. Their three children came along in time. Because of his easygoing and kindly temperament, Benjamin was highly regarded by everyone on the island. He was always ready when friends and neighbors needed a helping hand, and he was good at fixing anything that could be fixed.

At age fifty he developed a little bleeding from his intestine, and it just wouldn't go away. Benjamin ignored it for a year, but he had gradually increasing stomach pains. Finally, with severe pain, abdominal distention, and vomiting, he was forced against his will to go to the hospital with a completely blocked intestine. That was where Dr. Harry Byrd met him. Studies clearly showed a malignant tumor obstructing the large intestine. Surgical treatment was unavoidable. In the evening before surgery, Byrd went to Benjamin's room to explain the findings to him and his wife Rachel. The doctor described in detail the planned removal of a section of intestine to get rid of the problem.

Benjamin listened attentively and asked pertinent questions, which Byrd answered to the best of his knowledge. When it was time to leave, Byrd turned toward the door. Benjamin smiled his slow, easy grin and said, "Tomorrow, if you find that you can't do everything you hope to do, don't take it too hard."

Byrd, with his hand on the doorknob, was taken aback. In fact, you might even say he was shocked. It was his job to give as much confidence and reassurance to his patient as possible before guiding him through difficult times ahead, and here was the island man reversing the roles to reassure him. That had never happened before with any of his patients. Both he and Benjamin knew that the chances for cure were mighty slim because of the delay in treatment until the last possible moment. Early in the course of the disease, chances for recovery were quite good. Harry Byrd looked Benjamin Caldwell in the eye, and each of them knew that the other would make the best of a tough situation.

The next morning Byrd was depressed by what he found during the operation. The cancer had spread beyond the limits for removal, but he was able to gain some time and comfort for his new friend by shortcircuiting the obstructed bowel to bypass the growth. Rachel and later Benjamin, when he woke up, were informed of the findings, a painful duty for Byrd. For Benjamin and Rachel, of course, it was a thousand times worse. The bad news was accepted by both with considerable equanimity, since it was about what they had expected. The short term outlook was good. The obstruction had been relieved, and Benjamin rapidly improved.

Toward the end of his hospital stay, the island man said to Byrd, "What about Easter?"

Since it was September, Byrd figured that Benjamin's mind must have snapped due to the illness and strain. He responded, "What does Easter have anything to do with this?"

Rachel was sitting there smiling and gently cleared up the confused surgeon. "He means eastward, but it comes out eastard. He wants to know when we can go home."

"Right," said Benjamin. "Where we live, you can't

go any farther eastard on land this side of Europe."

A few days later they went eastard after arrangements were made for radiation and other palliative treatment to slow the cancer's progress. Byrd was pleased that things went along quite well for Benjamin for close to a year after his operation. At Christmas time, a heavy little box about six inches square arrived at the office by mail. Inside was a brass anchor and engraved on its shaft was the inscription "Eastard." There was no card, nor did there need to be one.

One morning during the following summer, Harry Byrd and Avis took a long ride, heading east, in their old Buick Skylark. Three hours later, they drove over the bridge onto Benjamin Caldwell's island. They didn't know exactly where to find his house except it was at Jackson's Beach, one of the several fishing villages on the island. They came to a village and stopped to inquire at the pier. Harry hailed a leathery-faced old man.

"Where might we find Jackson's Beach?" he asked.

"Yer in it," the old man said.

"Which is Benjamin Caldwell's house?"

"Right up there beyond the post office," came the reply. Sure enough, you couldn't go any farther east than the Caldwell home, on land anyway. It was a neat, white, clapboard house perched on a ledge, overlooking the sparkling blue sea. In the distance several trawlers moved slowly along, trailing their nets at the edge of a fog bank. Benjamin and Rachel were both at home, and they greeted Harry and Avis warmly. He was still getting along quite well, enjoying every precious day, he said, with his back to the fire in the walk-in fireplace of their living room. Even in the middle of July it never got real warm where they lived, and the fire kept off the damp chill. They went on a tour of the island, which was indeed as beautiful as Harry had imagined.

"Take a whiff of that air," Caldwell said. "If you could pump it into your hospital, people would get well a lot faster."

"They tell me florists don't smell the flowers after awhile when they're around them all the time. I'm surprised you can still smell the air," Harry said.

"I can smell it fine. If only I could bottle it, I'd be a millionaire," Caldwell said.

He showed them his weir, which he pronounced "where." He said, "Last week we took 400 'ugsheads of herring. Some of my friends use the new technique which is better than this old 'where.' They have a spotter plane out every day when it isn't fogged in, and the pilot can see the schools of fish shimmering on the surface of the water below. When they go into a cove, he radios down to the fishermen who go to the mouth of the cove and string twine (which he pronounced 'twoin') across it to trap the fish. Then, they go in with dories and spread a purse seine, gradually tighten the purse, and end up with a big net full of fish. It's a much more efficient method than my 'where,' but I don't want to start any long term projects."

They drove to the main harbor of the island, and Harry was introduced to Percy Young, who was working on the diesel engine down in the bowels of a trawler at the pier.

"Percy has a cancer in his innards that they couldn't

get out four years ago, but he looks pretty good, don't he?" Benjamin said.

A broad grin spread over Percy's grimy face. "Feel good, too. They told me I wouldn't live beyond six months. You doctors don't know as much as you think you do," he said. "In fact, one of them that told me that dropped dead on the tennis court last year."

"Well, Percy, you're the last person in the world I'd argue that one with," Harry said. "Personally, I never tell anybody they have so many months or years to live. It's too much like playing God."

Harry later looked up Percy's records at the hospital, which, strictly speaking, he shouldn't have done because he wasn't involved in his care. Sure enough, there had been a well-documented inoperable cancer. Must have been a slow grower, he thought, or else it's all that good sea air. You just never know about those things. As it turned out, Percy outlived Benjamin, but not by much. They both died within a year, too young.

Harry Byrd never saw Benjamin Caldwell again, but sometimes he thinks about him, especially when the afternoon sun shines through his office window and hits that brass anchor on top of the bookshelf.

The Native American

Francis Joseph Neptune and his wife Jean sat across the desk from Harry Byrd in his office, which overlooked the Penobscot River. The Neptunes had come from the Passamaquoddy Indian Reservation at the edge of the sea 150 miles away because Jean had a lump in her breast. They were both in their sixties and had been deeply devoted to each other throughout their marriage of more than forty years. Francis was obviously more worried than his wife. She sat there serenely with a smile on her round face. Her shiny black hair was parted in the middle, and a single braid reached nearly down to her waist. He held her hand tightly, with a concerned expression clouding his leathery aquiline features. They talked about her past health and the current problem. Byrd tried to encourage them, but he knew they would not be reassured until the exact nature of the breast lump was known. Nurse Bidwell escorted Jean into the adjoining room to change into a blue cloth examination gown, and Francis sat looking out the window.

"Look there," he said.

Byrd went to the window and saw a bald eagle soaring over the river. Its white neck and head stretched downward, with its white tail feathers extended, and its huge wings spread straight out. The eagle suddenly plunged straight downward and struck the surface of the river, then rose again with a three-foot, wriggling eel, gripped in its talons.

"It's a sign," Neptune said, "and a good one. I didn't know the eagles came here, so close to the city. I was afraid he had been sent by Glooskap to take my wife's spirit, and she would die from cancer, but now I know she will be all right. He only came here to fish."

"Who, or what, pray tell is Glooskap?" Byrd asked.

"You might call him a demigod," Neptune said. "He is the first man created by the Great Spirit. No one ever sees him, but he is around. He lives behind a waterfall."

"Which waterfall?"

"It varies from time to time. It might be Canada Falls, Screw Auger Falls, or Montmorency Falls near Quebec. It might even be Bad Little Falls. That's the translation of Machias to English from the Passamoquoddy language. Whenever anyone comes near, Glooskap just moves off to another waterfall. He knows everything that is going on, and when he does finally appear, it will signal the end of the world."

"I see," said Byrd. "Thanks for the explanation. I see the eagles here quite often, especially in the winter. Last winter when the river was frozen except for a few open areas of swift water, I saw an eagle flying after a black duck. The duck was so intent on escaping what was behind it that it failed to see the second eagle come in ahead, at right angles to the line of flight, and strike the duck from the sky. The two eagles tore the poor duck apart on the ice and then ate it. I couldn't believe that several other ducks idled around in a patch of open water, just looking at the unhappy fate of their relative not twenty feet away."

"Yes, ducks are even more stupid than people," Francis said.

"When the eagles flew off, three crows arrived and finished what was left of the duck," Byrd added.

By then, Jean was ready, and after the examination she rejoined her husband. Francis was visibly more relaxed, and she continued to smile serenely.

"We won't know whether that lump is benign or malignant until it's examined under the microscope." Byrd said. "Let's plan to get a mammogram and then remove the lump in the outpatient surgical department at the hospital with local anesthesia and a sedative. It won't be a bad experience for you, Mrs. Neptune, except for the strain of waiting to find out the answer. You won't have any pain except for a little stinging when the anesthetic agent is injected, and the small incision will be sore for a few days afterwards. If we get a good report, that's the end of the problem. If the tissue proves to be malignant, we'll need to sit down together again and discuss what else needs to be done. Even if the lump is malignant, there's an excellent chance for cure because the lump is quite small relatively. You did well to find it."

"I didn't find it. Francis did," Jean said.

"Quite a few ladies tell me that. I mean, their own husbands find it, not Francis." The Neptunes laughed. They agreed with the plan.

On the appointed day they rose before dawn and made the long drive to the hospital. They arrived at 7:00 a.m. for the scheduled 8:00 a.m. operation. As expected, the procedure of removing the lump was not a difficult experience for Jean. She never lost her smile. Twenty minutes later, the pathologist called Byrd with the news that there was no evidence of malignancy in the tissue removed.

The Neptunes were together again in the recovery area, holding hands and waiting for the report. "It's benign. Nothing to worry about," Byrd said.

"That's what I expected," Jean said. Francis just sat there beaming, and said nothing.

"Mrs. Neptune should rest here for a while before going home," Byrd said to Francis. "Will you join me in the cafeteria for a cup of coffee?"

"Good idea," Francis said. "I've been too worked up to eat or drink since we got up this morning." Francis had a couple of Danish pastries with his coffee.

"What kind of work do you do, Mr. Neptune?" Byrd asked.

"I've done about everything at one time or another–woodsman, fisherman, carpenter, mechanic, but I started out as a barber. I was the only Indian in the State of Maine with a license to scalp white men. During barber college I worked nights as a bartender, but that didn't last. One night a white man came in and ordered a Manhattan. I charged him twenty-seven dollars for it, and he was very angry. So I said 'What's the problem? That's what you white men paid us for the original Manhattan, half a cent for each acre.' I got fired for that one. Some white men have no sense of humor."

Byrd's opinion of the Native Americans was changing rapidly. He had always believed they were stolid, uncommunicative, unemotional, and inscrutable. That was certainly false. Not only that, but their skin was not red. Rather, it was swarthy and not too different from his own maternal grandfather who was a so-called black Irishman descended from a Spanish invader of the Emerald Isle.

Francis Neptune went on to tell him how the Passamaquoddy language and heritage were in danger of being lost. "At one time there were twenty tribes of the Abnakis in what was to become New England. Now there are only two, the Penobscot and the Passamaquoddy. There is only one surviving language, the Passamaquoddy, and it is threatened with extinction. The other tribes fled into Canada because of the wars between the French and the English, the settlers and the English, and because the settlers themselves pushed the tribes from their hunting grounds."

Francis' expression had been intense. Now the twinkle came back in his eyes. "One tribe was unaccounted for and seemed to completely disappear. That is the lost tribe of Fukahwee. No one knows what happened to them. Even today when our young men climb to the mountain tops, they look to the far horizon, shield their eyes from the sun in the west, and chant: 'Where the Fuk-ah-wee?'"

He continued, "When I was a boy, everyone on the reservation spoke the Passamaquoddy language. We are not really Passamaquoddy Indians. That is the name the Europeans gave us because we lived along the shores of Passamaquoddy Bay. We call ourselves Waponahkihik, the People of the Dawn. White men are Wapeyit in our native tongue. My mother spoke very little English. All she really needed to know was 'this basket one dollar, that basket three dollars.' The members of my generation are all bilingual, but our children have been learning only English. They watch the television too much and don't learn the language of our ancestors, but we have taken steps to preserve the language and history of our ancestors. Two men on the reservation have been working to compile a Passamaquoddy/English dictionary. Finally, they have received financial aid through government grants to complete this dictionary and also to publish historical data. These are now used in our schools to teach the children their language and heritage. We are also now teaching the children our traditional tribal ceremonial dances."

"What is the population of the reservation?"

"I'm not sure of the exact number, but it has gone up since John Wayne died."

When the Neptunes returned to Byrd's office for follow-up, Francis brought him four small books which had been published for use in the grades 4-8 bilingual program at the Passamaquoddy Indian Reservation School. One book was a historical novel entitled *Chipmunk - A Passamaquoddy Boy in the Revolution.* The others were *Book I- Amsquahseweyak Scicinuwok-First Indians, Book II- Skicin Eli PiluwikitIndian Characteristics,* and *Book III-Papahitomuwakon- Religion.* In these books the Passamaquoddy and English languages are printed in columns side by side. Harry Byrd read the books carefully. He was impressed by the man whose great pride and love of his heritage was thinly disguised by a devastating sense of humor. Neptune was determined to help his people keep their sense of identity and to be proud of who they are. In his words "Hollywood Indians always lost the battles, but this is one battle we will win."

A year later Byrd found out that Francis Neptune had been sent down to the hospital because of a heart attack, so Byrd stopped in to visit. Francis was lying comfortably and relaxed in the hospital bed. Lines from the cardiac monitor were attached to his chest, and a thin plastic intravenous tube ran into a vein in his forearm. Jean was sitting quietly near the window, smiling as usual, with the sun shining on her black hair.

"It's just a Wapeyit coming to visit one of the Waponahkihik," Byrd said, having rehearsed the words several times. "How are you progressing?"

"Fine, but I don't like lying here in this bed all the time," Francis said. "They doped me up and told me to lie quietly. This morning a pretty, young nurse came in to give me a bed bath. She washed my face and neck, arms and legs, chest and belly, then she passed me the washcloth and said, 'Now you do the rest.' So I took the cloth and started to wash her neck. She got all flushed and indignant for some reason. White people are very strange."

The twinkle in Francis' eye convinced Byrd that this man would recover well, and he did. After ten days Francis Neptune was back on the reservation.

Five summers later Harry Byrd and his wife Avis took a ride down to Eastport to see the new docking facilities that had been built there in the hope of developing that sleepy fishing village into a significant deep water port for ocean going freighters. They wandered along the waterfront streets and out on the dock where lumber was being loaded into a Belgian freighter. Then they walked to a shorefront restaurant and sat under an umbrella at a table on the porch. The sunshine was bright, and the sea air was clear and invigorating. Each of them ordered a lobster roll and a bottle of Heineken's beer. The rolls were piled high with large chunks of fresh lobster without the celery and lettuce space fillers that some tourist-trap restaurants customarily use. Afterwards they shared a big piece of lemon chiffon pie. Then they drove back over the spit of land that connects Eastport with the mainland. On their right was the Pleasant Point Passamaquoddy Indian Reservation, overlooking the bay and the green Campobello and Deer Islands of Canada. They passed beneath a bluff on the edge of the road. Harry recalled reading that in unhappier times Indian youths had been known to roll rocks off the bluff onto passing automobiles. "If you don't mind, Avis, I'd like to stop here and look up a friend of mine," Byrd said. She agreed, and they pulled up at the general store. "Where might I find Francis Joseph Neptune?" Byrd asked the storekeeper.

"He's usually at the museum over there," the man said, indicating a one-story wooden building about a hundred yards away. A red Pontiac Firebird with state legislature license plates was parked in front of the museum. Avis decided to wait in the car. Harry went in the door of the museum and saw Francis Neptune escorting two prim-looking, elderly ladies around the displays. An ancient birch bark canoe lay just inside the door, and rows of intricately woven sweet grass baskets were tastefully arranged on shelves. There were various types of moccasins, blankets and beaded buckskin clothing in display cases as well as primitive arrows, fishhooks, spears, and iron tools. Many pictures of past tribal leaders in ceremonial dress and Indian families at work and play hung on the walls.

From the conversation, Byrd gathered that the women were from the Ellsworth Historical Society. He waited until Neptune escorted them out the door. Then he said, "Remember me?"

"Of course, and welcome, Dr. Byrd," Francis said.

"Where's the visiting state legislator? I saw his car outside, but I don't see him."

"You may not see him, but you're looking at him. I am the representative of the Passamaquoddy tribe in the State government."

"Good. I hope you can help make some kind of sense in that crowd."

"I try, but it isn't easy. Let me show you around." He described the various displays and pictures. Then he called Harry's attention to an elaborate beaded and feathered head dress with a long train of eagle feathers. "This is a Sioux war bonnet. We have never owned anything like it ourselves. The Oglala Sioux nation loaned it to the Passamaquoddy tribe when we and the Penobscot tribe sued the federal government for the lands that were unjustly taken from us. The war bonnet is a sign of their strong support for our quest. Sioux—sue—get the point? The land where your home was built belongs rightfully to us."

"I understand you've won a pretty good settlement."

"Yes. Now we have both lands and money. Our people no longer live in shacks with dirt floors and no plumbing. We've built new houses for them and invested in businesses like the Dragon cement factory in Thomaston. So far, it's returned us a handsome profit. Now let me show you our next project here at the museum."

Francis opened the door to another room. There on the floor were about a dozen naked, pink, male and female mannequins, both adults and children, lying in a grotesque heap with arms and legs protruding in various directions. The massacre at Wounded Knee flashed through Harry's mind.

"What's this all about?" Bryd asked.

"I bought them cheap from a bankrupt department store in Boston. We plan to build an authentic, historic Passamaquoddy village here in the museum. We'll need people in it, appropriately dressed, of course."

"That sounds like a worthwhile project."

"Yes, and we'll need to change their color from pink to copper." Francis closed the door on the gruesome scene.

"You must come out and meet my wife," Harry said. They went outside, and he introduced Francis to Avis.

"I've heard a lot about you, Mr. Neptune," she said.

"Not all bad things, I hope," he said.

"On the contrary, it's all good."

Harry promised they would return in the future when the village was completed, and drove off, heading home.

"I don't believe anybody needs to be very concerned about the survival of the Passamaquoddy tribe's culture with men like Francis Neptune around," Harry said to Avis. "In fact, we may be damned lucky that we still own our own home."

The Lady from Hell

Andrew J. MacGregor was a down and out street person, which isn't too bad in the Maine summer, but in the winter a man could easily freeze to death. In fact, one winter, two people had been found frozen stiff, curled up like two fetuses in the womb. After World War I, MacGregor was mustered out of the Royal Army and left his native Scotland to seek his fortune in America. He was said by some to be a "Remittance Man," the name applied to certain incorrigibles in the British Isles who were sent off and received a monthly check from their well-to-do families as long as they stayed far away. If they ever appeared back home, the remittance checks would stop.

As it turned out, the fortune MacGregor was seeking never materialized. He worked long and hard as a woodcutter in Maine's North Woods. He had no close friends, never married, and he spent every penny he could get his hands on, mostly for strong drink and easy women. Eventually, a tall pine he was cutting fell the wrong way, and

MacGregor's back was never any good after that. He went from one job to another, always quitting or getting fired, mostly because he disliked people telling him what to do all the time. In fact, he disliked people in general. He lived alone in a rooming house and kept to himself pretty much. More and more of his time was spent in a hole-in-the-wall bar on Mercantile Square where there were no windows and the neon sign out front flashed "Danny's Bar and Grill." On the door Danny had a message, "No Chain Saws Allowed," to keep out troublemakers. Inside, Danny's didn't exactly resemble television's "Cheers." It took a while for a person's eyes to adjust to the dim light, and a pervasive smell of stale beer reminded one of the nearby college fraternity houses. But it was warm there, and the few patrons on stools at the bar, drinking Moosehead Beer, didn't usually bother anybody. Gradually, the bottle got the better of MacGregor, and it wasn't long before the landlord put him out of the rooming house. He wandered around the streets, spent time at Danny's, and at night he slept in the park near Hannibal Hamlin's statue, sometimes nearly as ossified as Hannibal. The long, narrow park was located next to the stream that flowed through town and joined the river along whose banks the town was built.

One night some youths, for no good reason, unless it had something to do with those funny roll-your-own cigarettes they smoked, beat up Andrew with Hannibal Hamlin's cane, which they had broken off. The police brought him to St. Augustine's Hospital where the Sisters took loving care of anybody who needed help, especially the poor, the downtrodden, and the unloved, just as they had been taught by Jesus. The hospital was a square, three-story, wooden frame building with patients on the first two floors and the nuns' living quarters on the top floor. The single operating room was on the second floor, and if a patient on the first floor needed surgery, he or she had to walk up the stairs to the operating room, since there was no elevator. When the operation was completed, the city firemen from the station across the street came over and then, accompanied by the anesthetist, carried the sleeping patient on a litter back down the stairs to the first floor. The firemen were always glad to help the Sisters because of all the good they did, and besides, it was pretty boring all day at the fire station, just waiting for a fire that didn't happen all that often.

Obviously, the hospital wasn't exactly a state-of-the-art type of place at the time. (It is customary now to use the term "state-of-the-art" instead of modern or up-to-date, just as it is becoming customary to say "I have the sense that" instead of "I think." Fortunately, the expression "at that point in time" seems to be falling out of favor so that people leave out the point part.) So, even though the hospital wasn't state-of-the-art at that time, the patients did very well, and they were overwhelmed by the loving care of the tireless Sisters who all radiated friendliness and good will, besides being highly trained professionals. In fact, they were so successful that in good time they were able to finance a brand new state-of-the-art hospital with three times as many beds. They could hardly bear to tear down the old wooden hospital to make room for the new one, and they kept postponing the demolition because they were so frugal and hated to waste anything.

While Andrew MacGregor was in the hospital recovering from his injuries of a broken nose, several cracked ribs, and various painful bruises, he was inundated by all that love, friendliness, and good will from the Sisters. This was a new experience for him. Even though he was a loner and disliked people in general, he was won over by the nuns. In their view his soul was just as valuable as the soul of the local bank president. It just needed more rescuing, which may or may not have been true. They knew, of course, that MacGregor's injuries were just symptoms of his basic underlying problems. So, instead of turning him back out on the street, they offered him a job as their groundskeeper and handyman. To everyone's surprise he took the job. They even fixed up a place in the basement next to the furnace where he could sleep. Fortunately, he had become somewhat deaf, so when the furnace came on with a roar, it didn't even wake him up.

Well, MacGregor's life was turned right around after that. He never went back to Danny's, swore off the bottle, and in fact, kept his promise. He dressed neatly, worked quietly without bothering anyone, and ate regular meals at the hospital cafeteria. It turned out that he had a green thumb. The scraggly, weedy lawn around the hospital was limed, fertilized, and treated with weed killer. Mac mowed it every week, and it gradually looked like a green velvet carpet around the hospital grounds. He planted flowers and flowering shrubs that brightened the whole appearance of the place with yellow, red, and orange blossoms. He ran errands all over town in the hospital's old Chevy pickup with "St. Augustine's Hospital" stenciled on the doors, and on rainy days he made minor repairs inside the building. In the winter he had the walks and driveways all shoveled, plowed, or sanded before anyone else was out of bed on stormy days. Dr. Harry Byrd observed all this with considerable interest. He had been on call that night when Mac had been brought in and had treated his injuries. Since Byrd was still young and underestimated the power of love, he had wrongly believed that the old man was a lost cause. So, Byrd gradually came to respect and admire the derelict who had rehabilitated himself, not to mention the admiration Bryd already had for the selfless nuns.

Harry had a serious lawn problem. He couldn't see the sense in hiring a landscape gardener when he had four healthy sons to do the work. His grass was pretty scrawny and full of broad leaf weeds and dandelions, even though the boys mowed it when they weren't off playing ball someplace. It had lots of brown spots where the boys were overgenerous with the weed killer. Byrd decided to get some expert advice on the care and feeding of grass.

One day, near the flower garden at the hospital, Harry found Andrew MacGregor for consultation. The old man listened, then spit a jet of brown tobacco juice with impressive accuracy onto a fat slug that was defoliating a dahlia. While the slug shriveled into a little, skinny, black cigar, Mac started a basic teaching course that Byrd obviously needed—when to spread the lime, turf builder, and weed killer, and how much to use. Later in the course, which was only about fifteen minutes a week, because they were both pretty busy with other duties, Byrd learned many things about flowers— how bright yellow calendula sheds its seeds on the ground in the fall, then grows from them the following spring, and how the lupine and columbine do the same. Mac showed him how to cut off dahlia stalks close to the ground in October, dig up the bulbous roots that look like potatoes, store them in the cellar all winter, then replant them in May. Also, since the dahlia bulbs multiply during the growing season, they should be separated from each other and not planted in a bunch the following year. Otherwise, you tend to get mostly leaves and not many flowers. Byrd was amazed to learn that although the winter kills dahlia bulbs in the ground, tulips, crocuses, jonquils, and hyacinths can stay right there through the worst of freezes and come up cheerful as can be in the early spring. In fact, his crocuses came up so early that they got snowed on and even that didn't seem to bother them. It wasn't long before Byrd's friends stopped reminding him that he had the worst looking property in the neighborhood. In fact, the grim-faced joggers and the fast walkers with their flailing arms even began to briefly slow down a bit as they passed by to appreciate Nature's beauty.

When Andrew MacGregor was well into his seventies, he asked Dr. Byrd to look at a sore place inside his cheek, right where he always carried the wad of "Red Devil" chewing tobacco.

"How long has that been there?" Byrd asked.

"Quite a while," Mac said.

On further, detailed questioning, "quite a while" turned out to be about a year. Mac had patiently waited for the sore to go away, but instead, it kept getting bigger and now was painful. By this time the cancer, because that is what it was, had a big jump on him, and the lymph glands on that side of his neck were suspiciously enlarged. The thing would have been curable in the beginning, but now that was pretty doubtful, Byrd thought. He admitted MacGregor to the hospital, and thorough studies didn't show much wrong with him except for the dumb cancer which was bad enough by itself. In the course of examination, Byrd asked MacGregor about a thin white scar that ran all the way across his forehead sideways.

"I got it from a German bayonet in World War I when I was one of the 'Ladies from Hell,'" Mac said.

"What do you mean, 'Ladies from Hell?'" Byrd asked.

"That's what the Huns called the Black Watch Regiment because we wore kilts and came at them with the bagpipes skirling. They found out pretty fast what kind of fighters we were. Starting back with Kitchener right up through Montgomery, the crucial battles of the English were won for them by the Scots. When a Hun came at me, yelling 'English pig', I didn't duck fast enough, and he lifted my whole scalp up just like he was a Sioux Indian. I got it all sewed back down again afterwards."

"What happened to the Hun?" Byrd asked.

"It was him or me," Mac said, quietly.

Next morning he walked up the stairs to the operating room, and after half his cheek and all the neck nodes on that side had been carefully removed, the firemen carried him back downstairs to his first floor room, which was easy because he only weighed a hundred and thirty pounds. Next morning Byrd went into Mac's room to check on his progress.

"Are you all right, Mac?" he asked.

"Well, if I was, I wouldn't be here, but I'm pretty good considering what ails me."

He recovered fast, especially with all that loving care from the Sisters. A month later he was back at work outside except when there was a cold wind that made the side of his neck hurt.

About a year later the cancer came back in his neck, which didn't surprise Byrd. Radiation treatments were started, and the lump began to shrink. Then one day Byrd was coming in the back door of the hospital when he noticed MacGregor mopping the floor with a regular wet mop. As he drew closer, he saw that Mac was mopping up some blood, and the blood was running down from his neck onto the floor.

"For Christ's sweet sake, Mac, will you stop that mopping and get in the E.R. with me," Byrd said.

"Well, I didn't want to mess up this clean floor," Mac said, looking quite peaked.

Byrd got him onto a table in the emergency room and put pressure on the bleeding place on his neck scar. In the operating room the artery that fed the bleeder was tied off, and the hemorrhage was controlled. However, it was downhill from there, and about a month later Andrew MacGregor went to his reward.

To this day the Sisters remember him in their prayers, as they do all people who are fortunate enough to receive their love, and when Harry Byrd works in his garden, he often thinks of the tough old Scotsman and smiles.

Cracked Marbles

One morning Jim Kestrel, the cancer specialist, asked his friend Harry Byrd to see Calvin Hunter, a ten-year-old boy who was being treated for leukemia. Just about all of the boy's surface veins had been used up, clotted by the regular intravenous chemotherapy that was being used to tide him over in hopes of a remission of the devastating disease. Calvin needed to have a centrally-placed intravenous line to provide access for treatment directly into his bloodstream.

That afternoon Byrd went to the boy's room at the hospital to meet him and explain the needed minor surgery to him and his family. Byrd was well aware that "minor surgery" is minor only when it is being done to someone other than yourself. Also, he needed to find out whether he could safely do the operative procedure with the boy awake, or if he needed to have him asleep. Children tend to be less cooperative under local anesthesia because they can't suppress their feelings as well as adults, who are just as scared, but have learned to cope with unpleasantness better. As Byrd entered Calvin's room, he braced himself for the emotional experience because, like most people, he hated to see kids sick, especially with such a serious disease.

Calvin was sitting up in bed with a Baltimore Orioles baseball cap covering his bald head. The hat was black with an orange peak, a little knob on the top, and an orange bird on the front. When Calvin turned his head, the cap stayed where it was and didn't turn with him because it was too big. He had on a blue johnny tied at the back, and his thin arms stuck out of the big sleeves. His mother was quietly reading in a chair near the bed. The most impressive feature about the boy were his large, calm, brown eyes, fixed steadily on Byrd. After Byrd introduced himself to Calvin and his mother, Calvin said, "My doctor said you'd be in. He told me they call you 'Painless Byrd.' Is that true?"

"Yes, like Bob Hope, who was 'Painless Potter,' the dentist in one of his movies," Harry said. His mother smiled. "How come you wear that Baltimore Orioles hat? I thought all Maine boys were Red Sox fans."

"Not me," said Calvin. "The Red Sox are a bunch of sluggers, just swinging away at the ball. No base stealing or bunts, and they never have enough good pitchers. The Orioles are different. Jim Palmer is my favorite."

"Funny thing," said Byrd. "My father took me to see the Red Sox play the Yankees at Fenway Park when I was your age, and he said the very same thing about the Sox. I notice it hasn't changed a bit in all the years since then. Of course, back then it was Lou Gehrig, Joe Dimaggio, and Jimmy Fox playing."

"You saw Lou Gehrig play? I saw a movie about him, and I got his baseball card," Calvin said, looking admiringly at Dr. Byrd. A box of baseball cards lay on the bedside table next to a stack of children's books. Also on the table was a big, pear-shaped brandy glass full of marbles of every color of the rainbow with a few clear colorless ones. They were of several different sizes, all round and smooth, but each one had many cracks all through it in irregular patterns. The afternoon sun, slanting through the window, shone on the marbles and reflected off them, and they sparkled with the radiance of precious rubies, emeralds, and sapphires.

"Where'd you ever get those handsome marbles, Calvin?" Byrd asked.

"My nurse, Penny Bolstridge, made them for me. She just takes regular kids' marbles and cooks them in a pan in the oven. When they get hot enough, they crack inside every which way, but they don't break," Calvin said.

"I notice kids don't play marbles as much as we did when I was young. One Christmas I got a nice bag of marbles, and a big kid won them all off me. We used to play baseball cards, too. Scaled them flat up to a wall, and the closest one won," Byrd said.

"We still do that," Calvin said.

Byrd decided that this kid was going to be very cooperative, and the "minor surgery" was done under local anesthesia. Calvin didn't complain, but he talked a blue streak during the procedure, both to Byrd and the O.R. nurses.

Calvin said, "I know my white copsuckles are

overgrown, and they eat up the red copsuckles. That's why I have to have blood transfusions to replace the red copsuckles and medicine to kill the white copsuckles. I just wish it didn't have to make all my hair fall out. Probably I shouldn't expect to live very long, but that's o.k. because I know God wants me."

Harry noticed that the nurse assisting him got pretty misty-eyed, and for a minute he had trouble seeing the stitches himself. This beautiful and wise child would never experience the many joys of life, but he surely was making the most of what he had. It wasn't fair, but no one had ever said that life was a mountain of joy. Afterwards, whenever Byrd was near the children's ward, he stopped in just to visit with Calvin. The boy did get a remission from his disease, temporarily at least, and went home feeling quite normal.

About six months later, Byrd sadly read Calvin's obituary in the newspaper. The boy had died suddenly, overwhelmed by the cruel disease process.

The next week Calvin's mother called the office. "I'm sorry about losing Calvin," Byrd said.

"He left a will," she said.

"What?" Byrd answered, surprised.

"Yes, he left his bicycle to his brother, and his baseball cards and glove to his friend down the street. He left you his cracked marbles."

Byrd wondered how it could be that a child, whose life never really got off the ground, could teach an experienced grownup like himself how to live—and how to die. He went to Calvin's home to visit and pick up the marbles.

He carefully placed the marbles next to the brass anchor on top of his book shelf in his office. There the afternoon sun shone in and made the marbles sparkle. Fortunately, Byrd possessed a generally cheerful and optimistic disposition, but every once in a while, when he had a tough problem and his patient wasn't doing as well as he had hoped for, his spirits sank. At those times he would sit at his desk and look up at the cracked marbles. His spirits never failed to be lifted.

The Ox Bow County Medical Society

Ox Bow County is a thinly populated, large geographic region of forests, mountains, lakes, streams, and scattered small towns. The people of the county are woodsmen, guides, sawmill workers, sporting camp operators, bush pilots, shopkeepers, truckers, railroad men, and their families. In the county seat merchants and tradesmen work along with a few lawyers and bank branch employees. The people are almost all hardy, proud, diligent, honest, and fiercely independent citizens. Not many of them have much in the way of worldly goods, but they have a wealth of natural beauty in their wild and unspoiled land.

In the third quarter of the 20th century the physicians of Ox Bow County were all solo practicing family doctors. They were few in number, twelve to be exact. Most of them were there because they loved their patients. They loved fishing and hunting almost as much, in a few instances perhaps more. Home visits were frequent. To serve the people, they traveled many miles over narrow, winding, sometimes unpaved roads. One of their members, Basil Swift, had been given free access to a handcar by railroad officials so he could reach patients in remote areas where some railroad workers and their families lived. In fact, he was allowed the use of the handcar for patients who had no association with the railroad, if he needed it. One cold night in the middle of winter, Swift and his helper were pumping the handcar along the track on the way to a primiparous, young woman in labor. They saw the headlight of a train unexpectedly approaching from the opposite direction on the same track. Swift and his companion swiftly leaped off the handcar into a soft snowbank. Their transportation was demolished under the wheels of the locomotive. They spent the rest of the night walking along the tracks to their destination and reached the patient in time for Swift to deliver a fine, healthy baby.

After Swift had spent fifty years of selfless devotion to his patients, the townspeople held a gala celebration in his honor, complete with a parade, speeches, and a giant barbecue on the shore of the nearby lake. Swift had attended the birth of most of the people in the parade and cared for them over the years when they were sick. First in the line of marchers came the members of the American Legion and the Veterans of Foreign Wars in their uniforms. Flanked by National Guardsmen bearing rifles, The Honor Guard carried the national and state flags. Behind them were the Ladies Auxiliary in their long purple capes. Next was the town fire engine, followed by a group of waving and smiling children on bicycles with red, white, and blue crepe paper strips woven through the spokes of their wheels.

Lastly, the high school band, resplendent in their maroon and white uniforms with plumed hats, marched along playing John Phillips Sousa selections loudly with a few scattered sour notes. The parade passed before the reviewing stand where the selectmen, the police and fire chiefs, the superintendent of schools, and the Congregational church minister all sat in folding chairs. In the place of honor were two chairs. Mrs. Basil Swift sat in one of them, but the other one, next to her, was empty. Dr. Basil Swift wasn't on the reviewing stand. Instead, he was marching in uniform with the high school band and playing the French horn. He had no problem finding a properly fitting uniform because he was slim and only a little over five feet tall. After the parade he climbed up to his place on the reviewing stand for the speeches.

Swift said, "Since this whole thing was in my honor, whether I deserve it or not, it seemed reasonable for me to toot my own horn." Years later, a lady in Orono wrote a biography of this much loved and highly esteemed physician.

The Ox Bow County doctors often were not paid by their patients, who managed all right when they were well, but couldn't muster up the cost of an unexpected illness, a new baby, or an operation. Everyone was treated with the same loving care whether they paid or not. The patients frequently found an alternative to money and paid their doctor in kind. A cord or two of cut and split firewood would be dumped on his dooryard. Fruits and vegetables would appear on his porch throughout the summer and perhaps a barrel of potatoes in the autumn. On one occasion a grateful patient, who was also a well-known poacher, unloaded through his doctor's cellar bulkhead and into the basement freezer the butchered parts of an illegally shot moose, while the unsuspecting game warden sat with his own pregnant wife in the waiting room above.

To a man, the Ox Bow County physicians held strongly conservative political views and were highly suspicious of central government. When an ambitious young Democrat with a charming personality and a sparkling smile was elected as their representative to the state legislature, the doctors had strong misgivings about him. Several of them invited him on a fishing trip, so they could listen to his views and inform him of theirs. The group was flown in to a mountain pond that was inaccessible by road and teeming with trout. They fished all day and stayed that night in a primitive cabin on the shore of the pond. During the evening the men sat around the woodstove and exchanged ideas about how the state should be run. The young politician's philosophy was radically contrary to that of the physicians. He was obviously a tax and spend liberal, and beyond their influence. While he talked at great length, they surreptiously loaded his drinks. By the end of the evening he was drunk and vomited into the stove. His perfect set of false teeth arched into the stove with the rejected stomach contents and lay there among the red hot coals. The good doctors put the aspiring politician in his bunk with a cold wet cloth on his forehead. They fished out the teeth with a poker and cooled them off in the water at the pond's edge. Next morning the politician was a bit green around the gills but able to function pretty well. He bravely flashed the winning smile that appealed so strongly to the voters in the recent campaign. It wasn't the same smile. The false teeth were all wrinkled up sideways.

The float plane returned to fly the group back out. The men picked up their backpacks and climbed aboard the plane. The politician could barely lift his pack off the little dock because his friends had thoughtfully loaded the large excess of trout above the legal limit into his pack in case the fish and game warden should stop them for inspection. Of course, they equitably redistributed the trout later.

The Ox Bow doctors were all native New Englanders except for two who didn't fit the mold. One of these was Solomon Grebe from the Bronx, New York. Grebe had visited Ox Box County on vacation and fell in love with the area. He escaped from the city and lived out his years in Maine. Grebe was well-accepted by both patients and physicians because of his devotion to the sick. They overlooked his strange accent and understood that perhaps he thought their accent a little strange.

Some of his mannerisms were annoying. Many of his sentences ended with the question "O.K.?" For example, "Take one of these pills three times a day for ten days, O.K.?" He repeatedly asked another question, "You know what I'm saying?" Both of these questions seemed to impugn the listener's intelligence, or attention, or both.

The other stranger from away was a Cuban doctor who had worked for the government in Havana. When the Batista regime fell, Manuel Diaz Tercel fled from the wrath of Castro's revolutionaries and didn't stop until he reached northern Maine. He too was devoted to his patients and well-accepted by all, but he had to overcome a language problem and improve his basic knowledge of English. The Mainers thought he talked as if his mouth were full of marbles. He compounded the language difficulty by greeting his Yankee patients in French. "Comment ca va?" The patients didn't care about his language problem because the most important thing in his life was caring for the sick, except, of course, staying as far away as possible from the Cuban revolutionaries.

In Ox Box County two small wood frame hospitals had limited facilities for treating uncomplicated problems, such as hernia, appendicitis, childbirth, simple fractures, congestive heart failure, pneumonia, and other infections. A few gallbladder operations were done on selected patients who weren't obese, but there weren't many of these. Tough problems were referred out to the city two hours away. The specialists to whom the patients were referred were those who understood both the Ox Bow County people and their doctors. An important requisite for referral was that the specialist take the same care of patients who couldn't pay their medical bills as those who could. Harry Byrd had no problem with that. One out of every three of his patients was a free patient.

The Ox Bow County Medical Society met four times each year. At the meetings they discussed problems in common, the latest statewide developments in medical and government politics, and listened to an educational presentation by an outside speaker. Annually, they elected officers of the society and the representative to the state society. Solomon Grebe was pretty much the permanent secretary/treasurer. All the members had taken a turn as president at least once because their numbers were so few and they had been members for so long. A search committee to recruit new members was unsuccessful. Young doctors entering their careers in medicine preferred to work near a modern hospital, and they shied away from the rigorous and demanding practices, obviously necessary in Ox Bow County. Eighty hour work weeks were the norm there.

Customarily, several specialists from the city, who had significantly helped Ox Bow County patients, were invited to the spring and fall meetings. They were charged $5 each to defray the cost of food and drink at the meeting. Nobody ever refused the invitation because the food, companionship, and ambiance were incomparable. The evening began with whiskey, beer, cola for the abstemious, and hors d'oeuvres of smoked trout or salmon as well as a variety of cheeses. This was followed by dinner, then the business and scientific portions of the meeting. At the spring meeting in June the main dish was freshly caught brook trout and sirloin steak. At the November fall meeting there was a choice of venison, moose meat, bear, and wild duck. Guests learned to be careful chewing the duck, for it was apt to be riddled with lead shot.

One spring afternoon Harry Byrd received a phone call from Charles Swan in Ox Bow County. "We'd like to have you come up to our June meeting and give us a talk," Charley said.

Harry could almost see and smell the pink-fleshed trout sizzling in the pan. "I'd be honored, Charley," he said. "What do you want me to talk about?"

"Whatever you wish. We'll leave that up to you."

"I've just finished studying all the cases of malignant melanoma in this part of Maine that have come through the pathology lab at our hospital over the last 15 years. Would that be of interest to the group?"

"Sounds fine to me. We're meeting on June 10 at Jim Gannett's summer place at Grindstone Lake. Just turn off on the left where you see the sign for the lake on Route 16. The sign has a set of moose antlers on top of it. About five miles down the dirt road, you'll come to Jim's place. You can't miss it, but if you do, you'll be in the lake. Try to get there about 5:30 pm. That's when we start."

"Who else from here will be going to the meeting?"

"Joe Gallinule, the cardiologist, Dexter Kite, the eye man, and Ed Kestrel, the orthopedic surgeon. Maybe you can all get together and come up in the same car."

"Good. We'll look forward to it and see you there."

On the afternoon of the meeting the four guests set out on the two hour drive to Grindstone Lake. Harry Byrd was in the front passenger seat, watching the green scenery go by and smelling the fragrant spring air, while Dexter drove along at a pretty good clip. None of them was exactly sure about the location of the turnoff. Harry spotted the sign with the antlers on top.

"There it is. Turn here, Dexter," he said.

Dexter swung the wheel hard left, and the car heeled sharply onto the dirt road. Harry pulled his arm back in through the open window. "Look there in the field! Wild strawberries!" Dexter exclaimed.

"I know, Dexter. I could have picked them with my

teeth. You nearly rolled us over!" Harry exclaimed.

They bumped along over the ruts and potholes at a more modest pace and soon came upon a big log cabin on the shore of the lake. Smoke was rising from the chimney. Several four-wheel-drive utility vehicles and pickups were parked on the grass in front. Jim Gannett greeted the guests at the door and invited them to pour themselves a drink at a table in front of the big fieldstone fireplace. Manuel Diaz Tercel was passing around a plate of hors d'oeuvres. With his mouth full of smoked salmon as well as the usual marbles, he inquired of Harry, "Comment ca va?" As he spoke, a little piece of fish was propelled outward between his teeth and landed on Harry's chest. Manuel leaned forward, balancing the plate on his left hand, and flicked off the errant tidbit between thumb and forefinger of the right hand.

"Bueno, Manuel. Or should I say, 'tres bien?'" Harry said.

"Either way. I'm bilingual," Manuel said.

Just then Francis Teal came up to Harry. "How is my patient Desiree Appleby doing, Harry?" he asked. Two days before, Byrd had operated on Desiree's breast cancer that Francis had detected on routine examination.

"Fine. All the lymph nodes were negative, and you found the cancer early, so the outlook for the future should be excellent. You know when I explained the options for treatment to her, she said, 'Take the damned breast off, Doctor. My ten kids used it for a lunch bucket, and it's served its purpose. Now I don't have any use for it.'"

"That sounds like Desiree, all right," Francis said.

"She's been rode hard and put away wet."

"Is it true what I hear that you've never sent out a bill to a patient in your life, Francis?" Harry asked.

"That's right. I just tell them what they owe, and they pay me at the office when they can. I can't be bothered with all that bookkeeping and paperwork," Francis said.

"There aren't many like you," Harry said.

"Hasn't done me a bit of harm. I have a comfortable home, plenty of food, my Chevy Blazer gets me around nicely, and Mary and I go out to dinner once a week at the Ox Bow Inn. That's all I need. I don't have a big stack of accounts receivable to worry about. Every patient I take care of is my friend. I know they will pay me if they can. If they don't pay, there is a very good reason, and that's fine with me," Francis said.

Just then Jim Gannett came by with an arm load of wood for the fire. "What's the news about my friend, Henri Bouchard, Harry?" A week previously Mr. Bouchard had collapsed while twitching logs out of the woods with his skidder. Gannett had diagnosed a bleeding aneurysm of the abdominal aorta and stayed with his patient in the ambulance on a dash to the city. Byrd had been alerted and took the patient to the operating room as soon as they arrived. The mortality rate for bleeding aneurysm of the aorta is 50% in the best of hands.

"I think he's going to make it, Jim. When we got in there, it looked like a bomb had gone off behind his intestines. We had to give him ten units of blood. His heart and kidneys are holding up in good shape. He's a pretty tough old bird."

"Of course, he'll make it, Harry. The only way you could kill that Frenchman is to cut off his head and hide it," Gannett said.

Byrd went outside where Basil Swift was broiling the steaks on a big charcoal grille, while the trout was being cooked on the stove inside the log house. The former handcar operator was now eighty years old and still carrying on a vigorous medical practice.

"I'd rather be out here in the fresh air than stay in there with all that cigar and pipe smoke," he said.

"Maybe that's one of the reasons you've stayed healthy so long, Basil" Byrd said. "By the way, I hear you're an expert cook."

"Well, I'm not sure about the expert part, but I do enjoy cooking. One of my favorite dishes is moose muffle stew," Basil said.

"I never heard of moose muffle. What's that?" Harry asked.

"The muffle is the nose. You've seen moose. They all have a huge nose. It's quite a delicacy if it's cooked right."

Byrd went back inside for another drink at the makeshift bar. Norman Merlin was pouring himself a generous shot of bourbon. Byrd quickly became captive to Norman's rather strange technique of holding his listener's attention by reaching behind him and firmly grasping the nape of his neck. This prevented escape quite effectively. Harry thought of the talking heads on the news analysis TV programs. Now he had become a listening head.

"Early in the war I was battalion surgeon for a tank outfit in North Africa," Norman began. "We went tearing around all over the desert chasing the Germans. There was always sand in our eyes and hair and clothes. We breathed sand and ate it in our food. One day this bedouin sheikh looking for help rode up on his camel. His eldest son had a bad eye infection and was in danger of going blind. Penicillin hadn't been out long, but we had plenty of it. I got permission from my colonel, who thought it would be a nice goodwill gesture, especially since we were having a lull in the fighting at the time. Off I went to treat the sheikh's son. The boy made a dramatic recovery, and the sheikh gave a big feast in my honor. I was seated on one side of him and the boy on the other, with all the other guests and relatives in a circle. We all sat on a big oriental rug and leaned on damask cushions in a huge tent. Steaming hot kettles of food were brought in and placed in the middle of the circle. They slaughtered a lamb for the occasion. None of it was wasted. The brains, stomach, intestines were all in this big pot with the rest of the meat. Of course, I stuck to the lamb's leg. All of a sudden the sheikh plucked out an eyeball that was staring at us from the pot and popped it right into my mouth. Apparently, the eyeball is considered a delicacy. I wanted to spit it out, but that would be an insult to my host. I rolled the damned thing around in my mouth for quite awhile. Finally I got up the courage and swallowed it, hoping it wouldn't come back up. Fortunately, for me, it didn't, but I haven't been able to eat lamb ever since."

Dinner was announced, and Norman headed for the food. Harry made a pit stop in the bathroom. As he stood emptying the bladder, a framed photograph of Lyndon Johnson, Jim Gannett's Democrat enemy, smiled down on him from the wall directly above the toilet tank. It was inscribed with a pseudo autograph 'Best wishes to my pal Jim from L.B.J.'

While everyone ate dinner, the noise of conversation was stilled. The trout and steak were cooked to a turn. There were freshly baked, hot buttered yeast rolls and a giant salad. The side dishes were mashed potato, boiled onions, butternut squash, and green peas. The members' wives had baked apple and mince pies for the meeting. All this was washed down with strong coffee.

After dinner the members and guests gathered in the big front room of the cabin. The sun had gone down, and the lake with the mountains beyond had disappeared from the view through the picture window, which extended across the front wall of the room. Members lit up their cigars and pipes. Basil Swift went home to escape the smoke.

First, the business portion of the meeting was held with Charles Swan presiding. The minutes of the previous meeting were read and accepted. Solomon Grebe gave the report of the secretary/treasurer.

"We have $80 in the treasury, OK? At the present rate we will, like the U.S. government, have a deficit by the end of the year, you know what I'm saying?"

It was voted to raise the annual dues from $25 to $35, and to increase the charge for guests at the meeting from $5 to $10.

"Does that bother you people from the city?" George Goshawk asked. George was known as the professor of angling because of his expertise with the fly rod.

"It's worth at least three times that," said Joe

Gallinule, the cardiologist, and the other guests nodded their agreement.

Solomon then reported that there was an application for membership in the society for the first time in many years. "His name is Roger Quail. He is a fifty-year-old orthopedic surgeon from Upstate New York, and he wants to move here, OK?" Solomon said.

"Does he like to fish?" George Goshawk asked.

"It doesn't say in his curriculum vitae," Solomon answered.

"If he wants to come here, there must be something wrong with him, booze, women, or money problems," Norman Merlin said.

"All his letters of recommendation are in. They don't mention any of those problems. You know what I'm saying?" Solomon said.

"Of course, I know what you're saying, but those letters don't mean anything. The people who wrote them are hand picked by the applicant. They wouldn't write anything bad. Maybe, you should call up the secretary of his current medical society. He'd be more apt to say on the phone what people won't put in writing," Norman said.

After further discussion and speculation on why this new man would wish to move to Ox Bow County, a vote was taken. The applicant, Roger Quail, was accepted into the Society by one vote.

The next order of business was election of the new president of the society. Roger was unanimously elected. Harry Byrd glanced at Ed Kestrel, who was sitting next to him. Ed's mouth was open, and his head was shaking in disbelief.

"They're all sick of being president," Harry whispered.

"Is there any old or new business to come before the meeting?" President Swan asked.

"Yes, there is a problem we must address," Jim Gannett said.

"This new government Medicare program has already fouled everything up. They pay me $20 for a house call, and the public health nurse gets $30. Now that just isn't right."

"There's a reason for that, Jim," Francis Teal said. "You go to the person's house, listen to his heart and lungs, leave a bunch of pills, and you're out of there in ten minutes. She goes in and gives a bath to the patient, does the dressings, teaches diabetics about diet and giving themselves insulin, helps new mothers with baby care, and so forth. She spends about an hour on her visit."

"Yes, but she can't do anything without my approval. I'm the boss," Jim said. "The boss should be paid more because of superior knowledge, training, and experience."

"Jim, you're a dinosaur," Francis replied. "The nurse is no longer the handmaiden of the doctor. She's a professional in her own right. You'll have to accept that fact and work closely together with these girls."

Gannett wouldn't subside, and he continued to protest until finally it was voted to have George Goshawk, their representative to the state medical society, bring a petition to that group urging them to work upward through channels toward at least equal payment for physician and nurse for home visits.

"Now that we have that settled, I'd like to introduce Harry Byrd, our expert speaker, who will talk about melanoma. You all know what an expert is. It's a man in a suit from out of town with a briefcase and slides," Charles Swan said. Everybody, including Byrd, laughed.

Byrd began his talk by showing a slide of a beautiful, smiling, young woman standing naked as a jay bird under a palm tree with one leg in front of the other to accentuate the curve of her hips. He thought this introduction might get the attention of his audience, which by this time of evening was getting a little drowsy.

"Melanoma can occur anywhere you see on this lady's anatomy, and a couple of places you can't see, namely the retina and the anus," he began. Then he went on, accompanied by slides, to discuss the hundred or so cases that he had studied. The age and sex distribution of the patients, location of the melanoma on the trunk, extremities, head, and neck were analyzed. The methods of treatment were discussed. These included the local excision of the primary skin lesion that was, unfortunately, sometimes inadequate, and regional lymph node removal which was a controversial matter. The long term results of treatment were obtained from hospital records and reports from the patients' physicians. These were compared with the results of case series reported in the surgical literature.

During the presentation Byrd noticed that several men went out to the kitchen to play poker, the glow of Charles Swan's cigar went out as he fell asleep on a chaise longue. After the talk George Goshawk said to Harry Byrd, "Harry, you're a good fellow, we like you, and you take good care of our patients. But, for Chrissake, the next time you come up here, talk about something we see once in awhile. In thirty-five years of practice I haven't had a single one of those melanomas."

Charles Swan, now awake with his cigar relighted, responded in Byrd's defense. "George, if you stayed in here and listened instead of playing poker in the kitchen, you might find some melanomas."

Byrd wondered about George's remarks, and later looked up the geographic distribution of the patients in his study. He hadn't thought of doing that before. Sure enough, the patients lived predominantly along the seacoast, and none was from Ox Bow County. Byrd speculated about why that should be. It was accepted, generally, that prolonged exposure to the sun's ultraviolet rays may lead to the development of melanoma. The citizens of Ox Bow kept their skin covered year round—in the winter because of the bitter cold and in the short summer because of the biting black flies and mosquitos. Along the seacoast, temperatures are warmer, and people had much greater exposure to the sun. The rays reflected from the surface of the water, doubling their effect. The ocean breeze blew biting insects away. Byrd concluded that George Goshawk was correct.

Today medical care in Ox Bow County has changed entirely. A modern hospital has been built there with the support of citizens, physicians, and the government. The up-to-date medical facilities attract young family doctors and specialists in a variety of fields. The doctors work with group coverage, having less arduous work weeks and more leisure time. The patients can stay nearer home for complex problems that require hospitalization. They less often need to travel long distances to the city for specialized treatment. The doctors of the old generation are no longer practicing medicine due to death or retirement. Charles Swan recently said to Harry Byrd rather wistfully, "The Ox Bow Medical Society will never be the same again."

Byrd agreed, and he thought to himself that there might have been a county medical society like it somewhere else in the country, but he doubted it.

The Seal

A dense summer fog had shrouded the coast for days. Then, a southwest breeze came up, and the fog retreated out to sea. Eben Abbott and his pregnant wife Nettie went mackerel fishing on that July day. A few white cumulus clouds with flat grey undersurfaces drifted along in the sky, and the blue waters of Frenchman Bay sparkled in the light breeze. In the background Cadillac Mountain and the surrounding green hills rose above them. Far to the east beyond the Porcupine Islands, they could see the edge of the fogbank. They were trolling along slowly in their old wooden fifteen-foot outboard motor boat. Eben was in the stern with a rod and line out on each side, while Nettie, who was great with child, lounged on cushions in the bow. She became quite warm in the noonday sun, so she leaned over the side to wet her kerchief and cool her brow.

Suddenly, a seal broke the surface of the water right beside the boat. The seal's smooth, dripping, black head glistened in the sunlight. The animal stared into Nettie's large, round eyes. She was so startled that she fell into the water beside the seal, which then dove and disappeared from sight. Eben cut the motor and quickly reached out to Nettie with his boat hook. He pulled her out of the cold water over the gunwale and back into the boat. She was trembling violently from the frightening experience, or the cold water, or both. He reeled in his lines, restarted the motor, and they returned to shore.

Two weeks later Nettie gave birth to their first child, a daughter. The baby was perfect in every respect, save one. There was a large strawberry red, slightly raised birthmark on her right hip. It was shaped just like a seal.

"It's a sign, Eben, I know it!" Nettie insisted.

"Oh, come on, Nettie. It's just a coincidence," he replied, but he wondered just the same.

They named the baby Celia, after her grandmother, not the seal. She grew up to be a beautiful, young woman.

Celia fell in love with Merle Newcomb, a young diesel mechanic, who worked in a boatyard at Southwest Harbor, and in due time they married. Merle was unhappy about the big birthmark that marred his wife's beauty, and he urged her to have it removed.

"You must never do anything to that birthmark, or I know you will die," Celia's mother warned.

"But, Mother, it's ugly, and besides, it aches sometimes," Celia said. "I want it off!"

The young couple made an appointment with Charles Crowe, the plastic surgeon who had recently opened a practice in Sunbury.

Crowe had problems of his own. He was the son of

From the desk of . . .

HENRY W. VAILLANT, M.D.

Hi Folks,
　　I enjoyed This
so much that
I got out *A Measure
of My Days* By
David Loxterkamp MD
about an F.P.'s life
in Belfast. Take a
look at it. Hope we'll
see you sometime.
　　Love H + J.

a famous professor of surgery in Cleveland and never quite lived up to his father's expectations. Young Charles finished medical school and trained to be a general surgeon like his father. However, he found the life too stressful with frequent life or death situations, so he took further training and became a plastic surgeon. He was not very successful in the university teaching hospital setting, so he moved to Maine where plastic surgery was pretty much a new field at the time. That move was unacceptable to his wife, who divorced him. Crowe was an avid golfer and tennis player. He joined the Sunbury Valley Country Club, which he saw as an opportunity to meet new friends. He got off on the wrong foot by making a pass at the local bank president's wife in front of everyone at the country club's weekly buffet dinner. After that miscalculation, he was somewhat of a social outcast. He also discovered that Maine women were so behind the times that they weren't particularly interested in face lifts, tummy tucks, or breast remodeling. One evening, while driving to the hospital for the monthly medical staff meeting, he got to thinking about his many problems. His attention strayed from the road, and he ran into the back of a parked pickup truck. His head struck the steering wheel with a resultant laceration across the forehead. He didn't lose consciousness, but everything was a little hazy for awhile. Instead of coming in the front door of the hospital, as planned, he came in the back door to the Emergency Department. Harry Byrd was on call that night. He meticulously repaired the laceration under local anesthesia, using spider-web-sized sutures.

"I guess this makes me the plastic surgeon's plastic

surgeon," Byrd said to Crowe, who was pretty embarrassed by the whole episode. Fortunately, the laceration extended along a transverse wrinkle on Crowe's forehead. The wrinkle was the result of a lifelong habit of arching his eyebrows upward which made him look somewhat superior all the time.

"That's a marvelous job, Byrd. I couldn't have done better myself," Crowe said, looking at his face in the mirror.

"As you know better than I do, it's because the cut is in a natural skin line. I can't take the credit for that. Good thing it was sideways instead of up and down or you wouldn't be so pleased," Harry said.

By the time Celia and Merle came to Crowe's office for advice, his forehead was well healed. After he had examined Celia, they discussed the birthmark.

"My mother was frightened by a seal just before I was born with this ugly mark. She is sure I will die if it is taken off," she said.

"Why that's nothing but a foolish superstition," Crowe said. "That birthmark is a collection of little blood vessels called a hemangioma. I can take care of it for you. Let's plan to remove it next week."

On the appointed day, Celia's operation was scheduled for 8:00 a.m. Crowe had informed the operating room supervisor that he would need about an hour and a half. The supervisor tentatively assigned Byrd a 10:00 a.m. starting time for his case, which was to follow. At 11:00 a.m. she called Byrd.

"Dr. Crowe is still working," she said. "There have been some unexpected problems. He'll be quite awhile longer, so I'm assigning another room for your operation."

"What's the problem?" Harry asked.

"The hemangioma turned out to be much more extensive than it appeared. In fact, it extends down into the pelvis and up under the buttock. He's run into a lot of bleeding. There seem to be large arteries feeding into it from several directions."

After eight hours of surgery and four pints of blood replacement, Crowe finally finished the operation.

Two days later, Celia had shaking chills and a fever of 105 degrees. Her pulse was rapid, and her blood pressure was low. Crowe asked Byrd to see the patient in consultation. The young plastic surgeon appeared haggard and pale. His hands trembled as he told the whole story to Byrd. "Her mother was right. She's going to die," he said.

Byrd found husband Merle distraught and pacing the floor in his wife's hospital room. Celia's mother was sitting in a chair with her knitting and had an "I told you so" look on her face. Byrd was reminded of Madame LaFarge in *A Tale of Two Cities* who sat at the base of the scaffold, watching the heads roll down from the guillotine. The only thing missing was a red Phrygian cap on her head, he thought. Byrd introduced himself and asked the family to wait outside the room. He examined Celia and found the incision to be swollen and inflamed. Then he took cultures of her blood and the incision and started broad spectrum antibiotics. After two more days, a virulent organism was identified from the cultures, and then the specific antibiotic to which it was sensitive was substituted. An abscess gradually developed beneath the incision and was drained.

To everyone's relief Celia recovered completely. Byrd figured that Crowe would have managed the problem well without Byrd's help. He just needed reassurance.

Not long afterward, Crowe joined a group of busy plastic surgeons in Florida where women were more interested in having their bodies remodeled. He said his relocation had nothing to do with the seal.

Lash Her to the Toboggan

Many people in the Boston area, where Harry Byrd grew up, considered that part of New England north of the New Hampshire border to be the subarctic. Byrd knew differently. He had been raised in the bitter, damp, cold winters of Boston where the east wind chills a person to the bone and blows dust, dead leaves, and paper litter over the hard, brown earth. Also, many Bostonians believed that northern New England was sadly devoid of culture. Boston, with its symphony orchestra, Museum of Fine Arts, ballet, opera, theaters, and universities clustered nearby was, of course, the seat of culture in the western hemisphere. However, Byrd had observed that most Bostonians rarely, if ever, patronized these readily available culture sources. They seemed to prefer basking in their nearness, as if they could absorb the benefits of this marvelous culture by osmosis. In their free time they went to the movies or the sports events at Fenway Park and the Boston Garden.

When Byrd moved to Maine, he was impressed by

the beauty of the Maine winters. The air was cold, clear, and fragrant with low humidity and usually not much wind. During the short days the sun was often brilliant in the clear blue skies. The ground was sparkling white instead of the somber winter brown he was used to, and the ubiquitous evergreen trees were draped with white cloaks of snow. On sunny February days he could walk on snowshoes through the woods to the sea and eat his lunch, while seated on a fallen tree with his back against the granite cliffs of the bold shore. Harry could feel the warmth absorbed by the rock from the afternoon sun, even though the temperature was in the twenties. He found that the severity of the Maine winters was not a problem. What did bother him was their length, which was two weeks longer on each end than it was in Massachusetts. The yellow forsythia was in bloom in April on Patriots' Day in Massachusetts, but not until two weeks later in eastern Maine. In autumn a killing frost was apt to devastate the gardens by early October, two weeks earlier than in Massachusetts.

There was an exception to these observations about the severity of Maine winters, between Christmas and New Year's Day in 1962, when a wild weekend storm just sat over eastern Maine for three days and buried the land in three feet of snow before the storm moved out to sea. Whipped about by the wind, the snow fell sideways instead of straight down, and it accumulated at the rate of three inches an hour. The result was exactly what the Bostonians believed were the standard conditions throughout the winter in Maine. Nothing moved for three days.

Fortunately for him, Byrd was not on call that

weekend, but as it turned out, an unexpected problem arose. His home was across the street from the hospital, which was situated on the banks of the Penobscot River and looked out over the river to the snowy hills beyond. He could rush to the hospital when needed, a big advantage for a surgeon. The disadvantage was that he was not infrequently called out at night when bad driving conditions made it difficult for others to come in from a distance. Naturally, he hated to get up in the middle of the night, but never refused when needed, although not without considerable moaning and groaning to himself.

During this big storm, an orthopedic surgeon, an obstetrician, a general surgeon, and a family doctor stayed at the hospital, as did an entire shift of nurses. None of them could get home anyway, and nobody could get in to relieve them. At the height of the storm, Byrd and his wife had a couple of martinis and a hot dinner. He banked the fire in the woodstove, went to the door to look out at the howling storm, and then turned in with Avis for a long, peaceful winter night's sleep.

At two a.m. the phone rang, and it was Robert Starling, the obstetrician. "Harry, Robert here, do you know Joan Walsh?"

"Of course, I know Joanie. She's our neighbor," Byrd answered.

"I know she is," Robert said. "We've got a problem. She's in labor and can't get to the hospital."

The Walshes lived a block up the hill from the Byrd home. Joan and Ed had five children who were close friends of the five Byrd children, and together they had great times, not to mention the considerable mischief they managed to get into. Just the month before, someone had opened the wooden gate to Mrs. Goos's nearby pasture and let all the cows out. Byrd was reading his Sunday paper and had a feeling that someone was watching him. He looked up into the big brown eyes of a cow that was standing right outside the kitchen window. To this day no one had admitted to leaving the pasture gate open, although the Walsh boys hinted it was one of the Byrd boys and vice versa.

"Do you have a toboggan, Harry?" Robert asked.

"Sure, out in the garage."

"Well, Jack Finch and I will try to get over to your house. Then maybe we can all work our way up the hill to the Walsh's house and bring Joan down to the hospital on the toboggan, or else do the delivery at home."

Finch was a young orthopedic surgeon who had moved to Maine from Pennsylvania that past year. He was energetic, enthusiastic, and very intelligent, but he didn't have much in the way of common sense. He was ecstatic about life in Maine.

"I don't even lock my house; it's so safe here. My dog can run free. The kids can walk to school. In one hour we can be at the ocean in one direction or at the mountain and lake region in the other. This is just a wonderful place to live and bring up a family."

Byrd considered Finch to be a little overly enthusiastic, and he was right as it turned out later. As an indication of Jack's shortage in the sense department, he had called police headquarters from the hospital. "This is Dr. Jack Finch, and I'm unable to get home from the hospital. I want you to send a squad car to my home at 78 Birch Street and bring my toothbrush and shaving kit to the hospital."

"Forget it, Buster," the dispatcher said, and clicked off.

Harry Byrd got out of his warm bed with encouragement from Avis, who loved Joanie Walsh. With considerable moaning and groaning, he pulled on his heavy clothes, overcoat, boots, and a stocking cap, even though he hated hats generally. He went downstairs, turned on the outside light over the door, and saw Starling and Finch struggling up the hill from the hospital, waist deep in the snow, which was still falling heavily and drifting in the forty knot wind. Robert resembled a tall, skinny Santa Claus with his big canvas bag of sterile instruments slung over one shoulder. The two men came into the house, short of breath in just that short distance up the river bank. They went out to the garage for the toboggan, and the three of them struggled up the hill toward the Walsh house. When they got there, they found a snow-covered police car stuck in the driveway. Inside the house Joanie was lying serenely on the couch under a comforter with her hands clasped over her large, round abdomen. Her husband Ed looked a little anxious, and the kids in their nightclothes were lined up on the stairway, peering through the banister. Officer Guido Casali of the police department was a basket case. He had come up to take Mrs. Walsh to the hospital and had gotten stuck there. Although Guido was a big, strapping, former high school fullback, he was terrified that he would be required to do the honors at a blessed event. The sight of blood had always made him feel faint.

"Guido, you look a little green around the gills. Why don't you sit down and put your head between your knees for a while," Byrd advised, and he did.

Starling unslung his bag of instruments. Then Finch piped up in an authoritative voice. "All right, men! Let's lash her to the toboggan."

Joanie rose up from the couch and planted her feet well apart to accommodate her ponderous abdomen. She grimaced slightly as another contraction arrived, and she announced decisively, "Nobody's lashing me to any toboggan." With that, she put on her heavy coat and hat. Ed had to pull her boots on for her because she couldn't reach down that far. Then she strode out the door into the howling storm while her rescuers stood there, mouths agape. She walked down the hill in the nearly drifted-over furrow the men had made on their way up. She disappeared into the hospital, followed by the men. Fifteen minutes later they had delivered a fine baby girl.

Byrd went back into his house on the way down the hill. He realized that he hadn't been all that much help, but he had tried anyway. His bladder had been sending him signals which were ignored in all the excitement, and suddenly he became aware of the urgent need to empty that overdistended organ. He stood before the toilet, unzipped his trousers, and fumbled with the front of his boxer shorts in a vain attempt to find the opening. Finally, it dawned on him that in his haste to dress in the dark, he had put his shorts on backwards, so he turned around, pulled down the trousers and shorts, and sat down like a girl in the nick of time.

The whole story of the great blizzard and the brave mother was duly and accurately reported in *Newsweek* magazine without, of course, some of the little details described above.

Officer Guido Casali had been thinking about quitting the police force, and his experience in the snowstorm settled the matter. He opened a pizza parlor and later expanded it into a very successful full scale Italian restaurant.

Dr. Jack Finch gradually lost his enthusiasm for life in Maine. Somebody robbed his unlocked house. His black lab disappeared one night, and Jack drove all around town looking for the dog. He spotted Sam looking out at him, tail wagging, from inside the glass door of Appleby's Paint and Wallpaper store. Sam must have wandered in there and fallen asleep behind the wallpaper racks, so that nobody noticed him when they locked up and left the store. Finch was about to break down the glass door with a large rock and rescue Sam when Officer Welch pulled up in his cruiser.

"Excuse me, sir, but what in hell are you doing?" he asked.

"I'm Dr. Jack Finch, and I'm going to break this door down to let my dog out," Finch said.

"What would you think about just calling up Mr. Appleby on the phone and asking him to come unlock the door?"

"Well, that's an idea I hadn't thought of," said the brilliant surgeon.

The last straw came when an unemployed woodsman exposed his turgid member to Finch's lovely wife,

117

Maureen, in the parking lot of the Shop and Save Supermarket. Finch moved his family back to Pennsylvania.

Little Dawn Walsh, who caused all the commotion by arriving in the middle of a blizzard, grew up to be not only a beauty, but her mind was brilliant as well. She graduated with high honors from the University of Maine and married a classmate who majored in forestry. He took a job as a game warden in New Jersey of all places. Contrary to what many Mainers believe, there are forests and farms as well as oil refineries in that state. Dawn became an accountant in an Atlantic City gaming establishment, and thus became one of the few people who profit from gambling. She was the sixth, and understandably, the last of Joan and Ed Walsh's children.

Tough Times

Moses Berry and Harry Byrd were sitting on the bold granite shore of the bay near a lobster pound that Moses had built in a cove on Partridge Neck. The morning sunshine was warm, and a gentle southwest breeze blew. Behind them the branches of tall pine, cedar, and spruce trees stirred. Below and in front of them several lobster trap buoys bobbed on the surface near their cork floats just a few feet offshore. A seal rose from the water, stared at the men briefly, then dove. They watched to see where he would surface again.

"The fishermen don't like those seals because they eat lobsters and cut down on the catch," Moses said. "Early every spring I see an old bull seal float past here, riding on a big ice floe on the incoming tide. He checks out the shoreline, then disappears under the water. About two weeks later, he reappears with his whole harem. The fishing must be good, for they stay all summer around that rock ledge you see sticking out of the water across there. In the fall they disappear again, no doubt headed south for the warmer water."

Harry Byrd idly watched a white dot far out on the bay in front of the mountains that rose in the distance. The dot gradually grew larger until he could see that it was a lobster boat making its way in their direction. He admired downeast lobster boats, designed and built for work and durability, yet artistically beautiful with their sweeping sheer, smooth lines, and gracious curves. As the boat approached, its engine could be heard. Periodically, the boat stopped for a while next to a buoy, then moved on to another.

"That'll be Sam Herrick," Moses said. "He's fished these waters in fair weather and foul for half a century. Those green and white buoys just offshore there mark some of his traps."

The boat was so close now that the crackling sound of voices from its radio could be heard. "That's the fishermen talking to each other," Moses said. "It's a little lonely out there on the water, so they chat back and forth a lot. They also keep track of one another, so that help can come quickly in case of trouble. The Coast Guard is great, but the base is always farther away than the closest fishing boat."

The boat pulled up to a buoy directly in front of the two men perched on the rock above, and the fisherman waved up at them. He was a rugged, stocky, older man with a peaked cap, plaid shirt, and a yellow rubber apron. His green rubber hip boots were folded down to knee level.

"How's fishin'?" Moses called out.

"Not good lately," Sam Herrick responded and smiled broadly.

"The fishermen always say that," Moses said softly to Harry. "It's not good when they catch a lot of lobsters because the price they get from the wholesalers goes down, and it's not good when the lobsters are scarce because they have to work too hard for a small catch. The price doesn't go up that much either."

Sam Herrick wound the rope line of the buoy over the motorized pot hauler and brought the wooden trap up from the bottom of the bay to the side of the boat. He swung the trap on board, opened it, and removed a good sized lobster with its tail flapping and claws waving helplessly in the air. He removed another lobster and tossed it back into the water. Evidently, it was too small to keep. He then removed several crabs and deposited them and the large lobster in a plastic container. Sam took a few menhaden, which the fishermen call pogies, from a bait barrel and placed them in the trap. He dropped the baited trap over the side, and its rope line ran out of the boat behind it, as the trap sank while he accelerated on to the next buoy. The boat turned away from the shore, and Harry noted its name stenciled in black letters on the stern:

TOUGH TIMES

Partridge Neck

"Sometimes I think I'd like to take up lobstering," Harry said.

"No, you wouldn't," Moses answered. "It looks fine on days like this, but there aren't many of them, and they can change in a minute, just like that," he said, with a snap of his fingers. "More often the weather is mean, wild, and miserable. It's cold, the wind is howling, or there's a thick fog, so you can't see past the bow of the boat. Of course, the fishermen know exactly where all the rocks and ledges are. They can feel their way around them just like you'd get around your living room in the dark without bumping into the furniture. Nowadays most of them are equipped with a Furumo radar, and that helps keep them out of trouble. Periodically, northeast storms roar in and wreck their traps. Of course, they have to make regular payments to the bank for the mortgage on the boat and equipment. Upkeep is expensive, so they have to be mechanics and carpenters in addition to everything else."

Later that summer, Harry Byrd stopped by Sam Herrick's house to buy some lobsters. Sam customarily sold most of his lobsters to pounds and restaurants, but he and his wife Ingrid also kept a saltwater lobster tank in a building attached to their home and sold lobsters and crabmeat direct to retail customers. Ingrid cooked and picked the meat out of the crabs. She prided herself on the fact that there were never any annoying bits of cartilage in her crabmeat. She came out to greet Harry. "What size lobsters do you want?" she asked.

"About a pound and a quarter. I'll take three," he said.

"Better take pound and a half. They're all shedders now, and with those soft shells, there's less meat in 'em."

"Right, that makes sense," Harry said.

"Another thing, how long do you usually cook them?"

"My wife boils them for twenty minutes," he said.

"That's fine for hard shells, but it's too long for

shedders. They get waterlogged and soggy. Better make it just twelve minutes."

While Ingrid weighed and bagged the lobsters, Harry looked through the open door into the house where Sam was sitting at the kitchen table. He was in his undershirt because of the warm day. Harry noticed that his hands, forearms, face and upper part of his neck were deeply tanned, but the skin he kept covered when outdoors in all seasons, namely on his upper arms, forehead above the capline, and neck below the collar line, was very white. Sam looked tired. He coughed.

"I have one of those damned summer colds," Sam said.

"Those always seem worse than in any other season," Harry said.

"That's about the heft of it," he replied.

Harry noticed two large burlap sacs of mussels leaning against the wall near the lobster tank with a little puddle of water under them on the cement floor. "Where do you get the mussels?" he asked.

"It's not far," Sam said, smiling.

Well, now that was a dumb question, Byrd thought. Of course he's not going to give away the secret location of his prized mother lode even to a landlubber who might possibly blab it to the wrong person. Let everyone find his own mussel beds.

"How's the fishing been?" Harry asked.

"It's been good, real good," Sam said. Harry was surprised, in view of what Moses Berry had told him. Sam wasn't supposed to ever say that. He paid Ingrid, thanked her for the advice, and left with his dinner for the evening.

In October of that year, late in the afternoon of a raw and cloudy day, a fisherman returning to port noticed a boat circling and circling in the lee of an island. He drew closer and saw the boat's name on the stern. It was "Tough Times." No one was in the boat. He radioed the alarm. Other fishing boats and the Coast Guard quickly responded. Many men spent the night searching for their friend and fellow fisherman. No trace of the missing man was found until the next day when Sam Herrick's body was discovered. He had washed up with the incoming tide on the beach of another island in the bay. It was speculated that perhaps his leg or arm had become entangled in the line, and he had been pulled overboard when he dropped a trap back into the water. This could happen even in spite of his long years of experience hauling countless thousands of traps. Or perhaps he had the sudden, severe chest pain of a heart attack and had fallen into the water. No one could survive long in that frigid water. There was no way he could call for help without his boat. Perhaps the last thing he saw before slipping under into the dark water of the bay was the stern of "Tough Times" pulling away from him.

Everyone along the coast was saddened by the tragic loss of another honest, good, hard-working man. Most folks knew or were related to other men whose lives had been claimed by the sea they loved and from which they earned their difficult and dangerous livelihood.

In November Harry Byrd learned that a memorial service was planned for Sam Herrick. The service was to be held on the shore of the bay rather than in a church. Sam was a God-fearing man, but he was never one to attend church services. On the morning of the appointed day, Harry and Avis drove out to the end of Partridge Neck. On the way they passed Sam and Ingrid's home. "Tough Times" was up on blocks next to the house. Harry parked behind a line of automobiles, and they walked over to join the group gathered in a field above the rocky shore. Sam's friends were standing in little clusters, some talking softly, others quietly waiting. Harry recognized shopkeepers, fishermen, truckdrivers, two retired ambassadors, mechanics, teachers, boatyard workers, lobster pound operators, wives, widows, a doctor, two nurses and the minister of the Congregational Church, a sweet, dedicated, devout, and compassionate woman. Byrd knew her to be a minister whose philosophy was to lead the members of her flock eventually through the pearly gates by good works and the love of God and all mankind, rather than to drive them there by preaching fire and brimstone.

It was an unseasonably warm and an eerily beautiful day for November. The air was still, the blue sky cloudless, and the sun reflected on the calm waters of the bay. The crystal clear atmospheric conditions caused the mountains, looming up across the bay, to seem much closer than the five miles distant.

At the opening of the service, a wicker basket with small, white carnations was passed around, and each person took a flower. Then, the soft hum of marine engines could be heard. A fishing boat came in sight from the left of the peninsula, followed by a procession of seven more boats, some rigged for dragging and one with traps stacked on the stern. The line of boats slowly progressed, then stopped directly in front of the mourners on the shore. Just then, a flight of six black ducks winged swiftly past in tight formation a few feet above the water between the boats and the shore, as if they had rehearsed for their part in the somber occasion. Sam Herrick's wife was in the second boat. She leaned over the side and carefully sprinkled Sam's ashes into the bay. Then, she dropped a green wreath of balsam fir on the water. The people on shore stood on the rocks at the edge of the bay and cast their white carnations outward toward the boats. The line of fishing boats turned and slowly returned to the harbor. The mourners watched until the boats were out of sight. Once again the broad expanse of the bay was empty except for the green wreath and white carnations, which could be seen drifting toward the open sea on the ebbing tide. The flowers looked like a flock of tiny sea birds swimming along together.

Harry and Avis Byrd turned and walked with the other people toward their automobiles. He became aware of the young minister walking beside him.

"I was deeply impressed by that service, Susan," he said.

"We all were," she said.

"But, I didn't hear anybody pray," Harry said.

Susan gave him a long, penetrating look. Then, she smiled and said, "The whole thing was a prayer."

Making the Best of It

Obviously, Monique Beauchemin's favorite color was purple. She sat across the desk from Harry Byrd in his consultation room. Monique was a tall, slim, good-looking woman in her mid-forties. Byrd noted that her hair was tinted purple. Her dress, earrings, eyeshadow, lipstick, and fingernail polish were all purple. Unlike most women with breast problems, she appeared relaxed and not at all apprehensive.

"Tell me about the breast lump," he said.

"I noticed it in my left boob two days h'ago when I was taking a shower."

"Ever had any lumps before?"

"No. I've never 'ad h'anything wrong in my life h'except I 'urt my h'elbow once."

"I notice you French people leave your "h's" off some words and add them on to others."

Monique laughed. "It's true," she said. "H'English is my second language. We French-Americans say things like 'I 'eat my frying pan and I hate my eggs.' I don't know why we do that."

"You do better than I ever would. Sometimes I have trouble just speaking one language," Byrd said. "You're married, aren't you?"

"I've been married to Pierre for twenty-five years. He's a h'alcoholic and drinks a six pack of beer h'everyday plus a fifth of vodka on the weekends. Sometimes he gets pretty mean and h'abusive. I married him for better or worse, and it turned out to be worse."

"Is he able to work?"

"Yes. He's a mechanic down at the garage."

"Did he come in with you today?"

"No. He says he 'ates doctors. They make him nervous."

"You don't seem nervous yourself."

"I'm not. I've learned to h'accept whatever 'appens and make the best of it."

"How many children do you and Pierre have?"

"Two. They've grown up and h'out on their h'own."

"Did anyone in your family ever have cancer?"

"My mother died of breast cancer. H'all the other relatives lived well into their h'eighties."

"Let's go into the examining room and see about that lump."

As Monique rose from her chair, Byrd was not surprised to note that her stockings and shoes were purple. She went with the nurse to change into a blue, cloth examining gown. The examination disclosed a worrisome, hard, irregular mass a half inch in diameter in Monique's left breast, directly under the nipple. There were no enlarged lymph nodes under her arms, and no masses were palpable elsewhere in either breast.

"We can quickly find out a lot about that lump with a needle biopsy," Byrd said. "That means taking a sample of the cells by inserting a fine needle into the lump, suctioning out a little tissue, and having it examined under the microscope. It won't hurt you because I'll numb it up with Novocaine like the dentist uses to work on your teeth."

"Sure. Go h'ahead, doctor," she responded.

The tissue felt gritty when the needle was inserted into it. Byrd aspirated some of it and spread it on a glass slide to send to the laboratory. An appointment was made for Monique to have a mammogram and chest x-ray the next day. Two days later she returned to the office.

"The reports are back, and it looks as if we need to do more about that lump," Byrd said.

"Is it malignant?"

"Yes, but there's no sign of spread from the lump anywhere else. The outlook for your future is good."

"That's what I h'expected. What do you want me to do?"

"The standard treatment today (*1960's*) is removal of your breast and the lymph nodes under your arm."

"Fine. I can deal with that," she said, smiling.

Monique underwent the recommended surgery. None of the twenty-five lymph nodes removed from beneath her arm showed evidence of cancer involvement. After the operation she did not complain of pain, or for that matter, of anything else. The operative site healed rapidly, and the function of her left shoulder improved with exercises more quickly than usual. A week after discharge from the hospital she returned as scheduled to Byrd's office for postoperative follow-up. She was wearing a tight, purple sweater and purple skirt.

"How do I look?" she said with a smile. She inhaled deeply and thrust her chest out.

"Like nothing ever happened," he said.

"I stuffed the left side of my bra with Kleenex," she said.

"After you've healed more, we'll arrange to have you fitted with a foam rubber artificial breast. It's called a prosthesis."

"Good. Can I wear it in my bikini?"

"Maybe not your bikini, but it'll be fine with a more conservative bathing suit."

They went into the examining room. "How are your shoulder exercises progressing?" he asked. Monique raised both arms straight up over her head without showing the slightest discomfort or limitation of motion. Examination of the chest wall and axilla disclosed that the incision was healing well.

"Good work. You're way ahead of schedule, Monique," Byrd said. Then he asked, "How is your husband adapting to all this?"

"Pierre used to sleep on the left side of our bed. Now he's moved h'over to the right. He says I look more natural from that side. He just spends twice as much time on the right boob as he did when he had two of them to play with. Would you believe it, Doctor, Pierre has stopped drinking.

Just like that. I thought he'd get the shakes, but he didn't. He's h'even started going to the AA meetings regularly."

A month later Byrd told Monique that she would need to return only annually unless any questions came up. "You should come back once a year for the next twenty-five years, then you can fire me," he said. This psychological tactic signified to her that she and he were expected to live at least that long.

A year later Monique returned, cheerful as usual. There was no evidence of recurrent cancer. "You are just fine, Monique," Byrd said. "How is Pierre progressing with the drinking problem?"

"He 'asn't touched a drop," she said.

"That certainly shows a lot of character. I hope he stopped being mean."

"Mostly. We did 'ave one little problem, but I took care of that. One day he said to me 'You know, Monique, there's a girl down the street who's been giving me the h'eye lately when she comes in for gas. I think I'll stop by some time and visit her.'"

"At least he's honest about it. What did you say?"

"I said 'Sure, Pierre, that's fine. Do whatever you like.' H'ever since he stopped drinking booze, he has three cups of tea when he comes home from work every day, and I fix it for him. So, instead of 2% fat milk I put milk of magnesia in the tea. He never noticed the difference. A couple of weeks later I h'asked him if he'd been to see that girl he spoke h'about. He said, 'No, Monique, I'm not that h'interested. I've been feeling a little washed out lately.'"

Monique smiled sweetly.

Life seemed to progress smoothly for Monique and Pierre after that. However, about ten years later, Harry Byrd noticed in the district court report of the newspaper that Pierre Beauchemin had been convicted of indecent exposure in the parking lot of the Shop and Save supermarket. The judge had fined him $250 and placed him on probation for a year. When Monique came in for her annual visit, Harry didn't mention this because he didn't wish to embarrass her. Besides, there could be two Pierre Beauchemins, but he doubted it. However, she volunteered information about the problem.

"Did you hear about Pierre getting fined?" she asked.

"I did see something in the paper. What was that all about?"

"Pierre 'as a problem with the prostate. When he 'as to go h'it's right h'away. He can't wait. So he keeps a can in the car for h'emergencies. H'according to him, he was getting h'out of the car in the parking lot and got the h'urge. He h'unzipped, pulled out his schlong, and then reached h'into the car for the can. If he'd gotten the can out first, he probably would have been h'all right, but he didn't. Just then, this woman was going by, and she started screaming. Pierre got tossed in the slammer, and I had to go bail him out. I went to court with him as a character witness. He told his story to the judge, but the judge wouldn't buy it. That was the most h'expensive piss Pierre will ever take."

One afternoon in his office Harry Byrd had a phone call from Monique. "Doctor, you said to call if I noticed h'anything h'unusual."

"That's right. What's bothering you?"

"I 'ave a pain in my side, and h'I'm h'afraid the cancer's come back. It started yesterday."

"Where exactly is the pain?"

"It began in the h'upper part of my stomach, then moved down to the lower right side."

"Any nausea or vomiting?"

"No, but I 'ave water brash and no h'appetite."

Harry knew that water brash, although it wasn't a term found in the medical books, was used by people locally and meant heartburn or acid eructation.

"Come right down to the office, Monique," he said. Further questioning and physical examination disclosed that there was right lower abdominal tenderness and muscle spasm. Except for slight elevation of temperature, there were no other abnormal findings.

"Monique, I think you have appendicitis. It has nothing to do with the cancer. We should go over to the hospital and get a blood count and urine examination to make sure."

That evening Byrd removed Monique's acutely inflamed appendix. As before, she made a rapid recovery with a minimum of complaints. A week after the operation she returned to Byrd's office. In the examination room he removed the lower abdominal dressing. The incision was healing cleanly. There was considerable adhesive tape residue firmly stuck to the skin.

"I'll just dissolve that tape with acetone and clean it off for you," Byrd said. "It would take forever for you to get rid of it with soap and water."

He soaked a cleansing sponge with acetone and

washed the skin. Monique had on her purple pantyhose with nothing underneath. Some of the acetone came in contact with the top of the pantyhose and the entire front of the flimsy material just disappeared over the crotch, groins and upper thighs. Byrd's eyes bugged out in amazement. Monique looked down and began to laugh.

"It's magic," she said. "You should see how red your face is, Doctor."

"I apologize Monique. I'll pay for a new pair of pantyhose. I've never seen that happen before."

"No, no, no. That was an h'old pair h'anyway. See, there's a run in the h'ankle."

Byrd was relieved. A litigious person might consider suing him for indecent assault or something. Not only that, but if OSHA ever got wind of it, he might be fined for keeping hazardous chemicals in the office. When he thought about it later, he realized what had happened. The pantyhose are made of synthetic nylon acetate and therefore, are soluble in acetone.

Twenty-five years after the breast cancer treatment, Monique Beauchemin was in excellent health. However, she had some concerns about her home situation.

"I'm afraid Pierre is getting h'Alzheimer's disease."

"What makes you think that?" Byrd asked.

"Well, the h'other morning he was looking all h'over the bedroom for 'is socks. I 'ad to tell him that they were on his feet."

"Maybe he was just still sleepy. I've been known to put on two different colored socks myself."

"H'another thing. He's stopped being 'orny. So I

said, 'Pierre, h'aren't you h'interested in sex h'anymore?' And he said, 'Oh, I'm still h'interested, but I can't remember why?'"

"That could be just a sign of aging. The old hormones slow down some eventually you know." Byrd thought that perhaps Pierre was showing early signs of Alzheimer's disease, but knowing Monique, he was sure that whatever happened, she would make the best of it, just as she always had.

The Gardener

One cool, sunny morning in the summer Harry Byrd set out on his regular walk. He preferred walking to jogging because the walker can stop to smell the flowers and listen to the songbirds in the trees. The jogger gains the benefit of greater physical stimulation and a certain euphoria but goes past everything too fast; once he starts out, he can't stop and misses a lot along the way.

When Byrd walked past the house of Amy Hardy Folsom, he saw her coming from behind the house. She was dressed in bib overalls over a flower-patterned blouse. There were grass stains on the knees of the overalls. In one hand she was carrying a clay flower pot and in the other, a green trowel.

"Come see my garden," she called out to him. Amy was a slim, cheerful, vigorous lady of eighty-five years who lived alone in her neatly-kept, small, white house. It had been built close to the road for easy access through the winter snow and ice. On either side, the nearest house was

200 yards or more away. Behind the house was a flower garden, shaped like the letter 'C' with its open base along the house and a green lawn in the hollow part of the 'C'. In the middle of the lawn there was a round, white wrought iron table with a big, yellow and white striped umbrella sticking up through a hole in the middle of it. Several comfortable white chairs were arranged near the table. The garden was in full bloom. It was carefully arranged, with the taller plants along the back and dwarf types on the front border. There wasn't a weed in it.

Byrd knew this garden was the love of Amy's life. For six months of the year, except when it rained too hard, she spent most of her waking hours tending it with loving care. "My spring flowers have gone by, of course," Amy said, as she escorted Byrd around the garden. "I start as soon as the mud season ends in early May. First, the crocuses come up, then the daffodils, jonquils, hyacinths, and tulips, along with my rhododendrons. Over there you see the azaleas. Even though they're the hardy type, they get winter killed every few years, and I have to replace them. Azaleas are best suited for the warmer climates down in Virginia, Georgia, and the Carolinas, of course, where the winters are mild, and the spring season is two months ahead of ours, but then it gets too hot there in the summer for me. Around Memorial Day I plant my geraniums, petunias, marigolds, and salvia, and the impatiens are there in the shade, which they prefer. They all blossom right through summer 'til the killing frost in October. The lupine, peonies, and columbine blossom by the end of June. Then, gradually, those daisies, lilies, dahlias, delphinium, and tall phlox come in, followed by the

Canterbury Bells, Sweet William, snapdragons and Johnny Jump-Ups. Finally, in late summer the chrysantheums, monkshood, sedum, bachelor buttons and cosmos bloom. Of course, all the primary colors are represented, but I especially love the various shades and blending of colors like the pale pink astilbe, deep pink Canterbury Bells, and rusty pink sedum. Then, there are varieties of red with the scarlet poppies, burgundy snapdragons and crimson dahlias. Notice the change from sky blue violas to blue campanulas, dark blue monkshoods, deep blue lupines, steel blue globe thistles, then lavender blue cranesbill, lavender aster and purple petunias."

After the tour around the garden, Amy brought a pitcher of iced tea and two tumblers from the house. The two of them sat by the table under the umbrella, while the flowers around them nodded and swayed in the breeze. A hummingbird suddenly flew by into the garden. Its wings moved so rapidly they were a blur and made a whirring sound. The bird hovered like a miniature helicopter over an orange tiger lily and plunged its long beak into the center of the flower to drink in its nectar.

"They're attracted to the brightest colored flowers," Amy said.

"Do you grow any vegetables, Amy?" Harry asked.

"My brother-in-law, Ralph, says he will never grow anything he can't eat. He just doesn't know how much he is missing," Amy said. "I always did have a vegetable garden until a few years back, but it became too much of a battle. Every spring Joe Carson tilled the garden for me with his big tractor, and I planted it. First, the crows came and dug up the sprouting corn to get at the kernels underneath. Then those striped beetles came all the way from Colorado and defoliated my potato plants. I hate to use pesticides in the garden. You never know what bad things they do to the vegetables when you eat them. Every morning I was out picking off beetles and putting them in a covered mayonnaise jar, but they still kept ahead of me. Those fat, ugly slugs ruined the lettuce, and the field mice reached up and ate the lower ends of the bush beans as they hung down. At night the deer came up through the woods and cleaned the beets, carrots, and what was left of the beans right off level with the ground. Then, just as the corn ripened and my mouth was watering for it, in came the raccoons. They picked the ears right off the stalks with their little fingers and stripped the kernels from every cob, just as neat as can be. So I gave up, and now there are only those tomatoes you see at the back of the garden, and of course, the herbs. I grow chives, thyme, sweet basil, and some mint."

Amy rose from her chair and picked a few mint leaves which she crumpled up and put into their glasses of tea. "Try it. It tastes good," she said. "Of course, it's even better in spring water and a little bourbon but not until the sun gets over the yard-arm."

"You must get sad when winter comes, and all this beauty shrivels up and disappears," Byrd said.

"Well, yes, in a way I do get a little sad, but winter is beautiful in another way with the white ground, the frost designs on the windows, and the layers of snow on the evergreen trees. I keep busy. That's when I make my afghans, quilts, and hooked rugs. I love to knit, so I do sweaters, hats, and mittens for the children of friends and send some off to the grandchildren. The members of the Women's Guild at the church run craft and bake sales. We ladies bring in our fresh baked bread, yeast rolls, doughnuts, brownies, fudge, and chocolate chip cookies. They all get snapped up pretty fast. The winter goes by, but awfully slowly. It isn't the severity I mind but the length of it. Around Boston the forsythia blooms mid-April, but it's usually two weeks later here. The crocuses come up here in April, then often get covered by a late snowstorm. They don't seem to mind, though. The snow melts quickly, and then they are just as perky as ever. I must say, it's exciting when the Burpee's seed catalogue shows up in my mailbox. It may be only the end of February, but those flowers in their natural colors on every page just announce to the world that spring is coming. Mr. Burpee, who founded the company, has gone now, rest his soul. He had a wonderful love of gardening that I read about in the newspaper. He said something like this, 'If you want to be happy for an hour, get drunk. If you want to be happy for a weekend, get married. If you want to be happy for a whole week, kill your pig and eat it. But if you want to be happy all your life, become a gardener.'"

Harry Byrd finished his mint tea, thanked his hostess, and continued his walk. Amy made him promise to stop by again, which he did late in the summer when the days were getting shorter, and a hint of a chill was in the wind, and the crickets were chirping in the fields.

"I need your advice," Amy said. "I realize that you are a cutting surgeon, and this is not in your line, but maybe you can steer me in the right direction."

"You know I'll do what I can to help, Amy," Harry said. "Tell me what ails you."

"Well, lately, when I work in the garden, I get light-headed, and my breath comes in short pants. At first I shrugged it off, but it's gradually getting worse."

"It sounds like you may have a little problem with your heart, Amy. There are lots of things that can be done to help that sort of trouble."

"Like what?" she asked.

"Usually medication, like digitalis. That's a derivative of one of your plants, the foxglove, and it's used to strengthen the heart. I'll arrange an appointment for you with a friend of mine, Billy Killdeer, who's a good cardiologist. He used to be a medical school professor in New York, but he got fed up with the big city and medical politics, so he moved up here for the better life."

"Good, I wish you'd do that," she said.

Amy went to see Doctor Killdeer at the appointed time. He listened to her story, examined her, and arranged for studies, including electrocardiogram, stress test, echocardiogram, and cardiac catheterization. Afterward, Killdeer called Byrd to report his findings.

"Amy has a tight narrowing of the aortic valve of her heart," he said. "She could die suddenly at any time now, especially with physical exertion. Medication probably won't help much. I hate to say this, but she may be a candidate for an aortic valve replacement."

"My God, Billy, she's eighty-five years old!" Harry said.

"I know, but her body and certainly her mind are

twenty years younger than her age. What I'd like to do is send her to the heart surgeons in Boston and get their opinion about it. The treatment of heart disease is a whole new ballgame nowadays, and as you know, those people down there are pioneers in the surgical treatment of it."

Harry went to see Amy in the hospital and pulled up a chair next to her bed. Her children had come back from away because of their mother's health problem. In Maine, "away" can be anywhere from New Hampshire to Afghanistan. In this instance, one of the four children came from Alaska and the rest from various other states. Two of them thought the idea of heart surgery for their mother was terrible, and the other two said that perhaps she should at least consider it. All the neighbors up and down the road back home and friends at church got word, of course, about Amy's situation, and they all had an opinion. Again, there was about an equal division between those who favored and those who opposed the idea of surgery.

"What do you think about all this, Amy?" Harry asked.

"Well, I can't just go according to a vote by all my relatives and friends, Harry. I've had a good life and a long one. My first marriage was for love. Howard Hardy and I had a wonderful life together. He was a school teacher and full of life with a great sense of humor. I'll never forget our Sunday picnics. A group of families would get together each week, and after church services we all set out with our picnic baskets full of crabmeat sandwiches and fried chicken and sliced cucumbers, pickles, and deviled eggs. There were thermos jugs full of coffee and bottles of soda pop in the cooler for the children. Only one person would know where we were going. We all took turns being the leader. Five or six Fords and Studebakers and Hudsons followed the leader. We ended up at a lake or the seashore and sometimes the mountains. When Howard was the leader, he always picked out the best picnic places, with marvelous views and nobody else around to bother our group. After he died, I waited a decent period of time, and then married Roger Folsom. This time it was more for security reasons. Howard didn't leave much in the way of worldly goods. Roger owned a coal and oil business. He was good to me, but he was somewhat stodgy and humorless. You might even say he was a rather sour individual. In fact, there were those who said he behaved as if he was sitting on a lemon wedge. When he died, I was financially comfortable, with my home all paid for and of course, I had the garden. Your friend, Doctor Killdeer, told me that I couldn't work in my garden anymore. I'm supposed to just sit around the house like an old lady, which, of course, I am. There is a risk to having the surgery, but if it is successful, there would be no limitation of activity. I could work in the garden again. My decision is made. If I can't work in my garden, I would rather die on the operating table and have it done with. Now, please explain to me just exactly what they do."

"Here's the problem. The heart is a pump built of muscle fibers. Your heart is strong, and the coronary arteries that supply the heart muscle itself with blood are clear and open. However, the valve at your heart's outlet, which allows blood to be pumped out into the body's circulation, is defective," Byrd paused. Amy listened intently.

"The valve has become very narrow. It's called "stenosis." No matter how hard your heart pumps, it can't push enough blood through that shrunken and constricted valve. When you exert yourself, your body, of course, needs more blood flow, but that narrow outlet prevents it. Nowadays what can be done is to put in a new valve."

"How do they do that?"

"Your heart is approached through an incision down the middle of the chest in front."

"How do they get through the breast bone."

"With an electric saw."

"How gross. I've read about those old Aztec priests who stood on top of a pyramid and plucked out the hearts of their living sacrificial victims. I'll bet they would have loved to get a hold of one of those electric saws."

"It is gross, but once inside, it's an extremely delicate operation. First, your heart beat is stopped. They can't work on it when it's bouncing around."

"How is that done?"

"Your heart is bathed in ice water and a special chemical solution. Meanwhile, a mechanical pump and oxygenator off to one side is connected to your body as a temporary substitute for your heart. Blood continues to flow to your brain and vital organs in the rest of your body, but not through your heart, which is by-passed. Then, the malfunctioning valve is taken out, and a new one is sewed in its place. Your heart is warmed up again and resumes its beat. The temporary pump is disconnected. Your breast bone is secured back together, and the skin incision is closed."

"Well, there. Isn't that something!" Amy exclaimed. She was admitted to the Peter Bent Brigham Hospital. A team of cardiologists and cardiac surgeons carefully evaluated the patient and her studies. They agreed that the risk for surgery was reasonable, although Amy would be the oldest patient ever in their highly successful heart surgery program.

Amy didn't die on the operating table. Her recovery was rapid and impressive. She endeared herself to all her doctors and nurses who were deeply touched by her toughness, resiliency, and her cheerful, uncomplaining attitude. When she returned to her home for convalescence after surgery, Harry Byrd stopped by to visit.

"Your family and all your friends are rejoicing, Amy. You got along better than most people. That was certainly the right decision you made," he said.

"That's what they all told me up there at the hospital," she said. "There is one thing that you didn't explain to me, and they did later. You said the surgeons would put in a new valve."

"That's right, I did," he said.

"Well, it wasn't new. It was secondhand. They told me they took it out of a pig's heart," she said.

"As long as it works well, and it does, what difference does it make?" he said. "There's no reason for you to get all fussed up about it."

"I suppose it doesn't make a damn bit of difference, except to the pig. I have an idea he would have taken a dim view of the whole idea. In any event, I'd appreciate if it you don't mention where it came from to my friends."

When spring came, Amy was back in her garden, which blossomed more beautifully than ever that summer. She continued her full activity without any symptoms for another ten years. Then, one night in the autumn she slipped away in her sleep at age 95. The next summer Harry Byrd stopped by on one of his morning walks to look at Amy's garden. No annuals had been planted, of course, and the perennials were choked off by invading weeds and brambles. The symphony of color no longer existed because its conductor had gone to an even more beautiful but unearthly garden that knows no winter.

The Ulcerogenic Cows

J. Hartwell Cripps was brought by ambulance to the hospital in the night because of a bloody flux. Without apparent warning he had felt faint, passed a large, black stool, and vomited half a basinful of bright red blood. Dr. Byrd met Cripps in the emergency room and noted that he was a tall, slim, rather handsome, silver-grey haired man of about fifty years. His shirt, trousers, shoes, and socks were black. When Byrd and the nurse helped him out of his clothes and into a hospital johnny, they saw that his undershirt and jockey shorts were also black, contrasting with his pale white skin. Even his lips and nailbeds were white. His blood pressure was low, and his pulse was weak and rapid. A blood sample was drawn for analysis, coagulation studies, typing, and matching with compatible blood. Intravenous lines were placed for fluid and blood replacement. Meanwhile, Byrd took a rapid history and examined the patient.

"Have you been having any pain, Mr. Cripps?"

149

"None. I just feel weak and all gone."

"Have you ever had any bleeding before, or do you bruise easily?"

"No."

"Do you drink alcohol much?"

"Never."

"Take any medicines, aspirin for instance?"

"No."

"What illnesses have you had in the past?"

"None. I've always been healthy."

"How about heartburn?"

"Oh, sure. Heartburn wakes me up at night ever since I got involved with those damned cows. I'm a dairy farmer."

"Does it bother you in the daytime?"

"Usually about an hour after I eat."

"Have you seen a doctor about it?"

"No, I just take 'Rolaids' or drink some milk. God knows there's always plenty of milk around. After a while the burning goes away."

That was the clue Byrd needed. He found nothing else of significance in the history and examination. "Mr. Cripps, it looks as though you have a bleeding ulcer," he said. "We'll need some studies to be sure. An ulcer is like a cigarette hole burned in a blanket. Stomach acid burns a hole in the lining of a person's stomach or more often, the part of the intestine just beyond the outlet of the stomach called the duodenum. Sometimes, the ulcer erodes right into a blood vessel in its base and that causes the bleeding."

"So, what do you do about it?" Cripps asked.

"You've lost a lot of blood, so we run blood in through your veins faster than you lose it, and in the meantime we do things to heal the ulcer. We give you medicine to block the acid and coat the ulcer. You'll also need sedatives to relax you. Rest for the mind and body is very important."

"What if it doesn't stop bleeding?"

"Usually, it does stop, but if it doesn't, then you'll need an operation to control it."

"Who would do the operation?"

"I would, unless you'd prefer another surgeon."

"I don't know any other surgeons, so I'll have to keep you."

"If it's any reassurance, I've never taken care of anybody with this problem who didn't come through the operation all right, and that's over a hundred people."

"I'd hate to be the first one you lose. What causes ulcers anyway?"

"Nobody really knows, but there are plenty of theories. Too much acid is the basic thing." *(now known to be caused by a specific bacteria)*

"It's those damned cows. I just know it," Cripps asserted. Byrd made a mental note to inquire into that interesting theory later when the situation was more stable. In the next twenty-four hours, six pints of blood were replaced. Daniel Curlew, the gastroenterologist, looked down into Cripps' stomach and duodenum with his periscope-like flexible endoscope. Sure enough, there was a round ulcer crater just beyond the stomach in the duodenum, and in its base an artery that looked like the end of a piece of spaghetti with a clot on its surface. The bleeding stopped initially, but then, it recurred vigorously with another drop in blood pressure, fast pulse rate, and the passage of voluminous, burgundy wine-colored stools. No doubt the clot on the piece of spaghetti had come loose. By this time it was late in the evening, and it happened to be Christmas Eve. Harry Byrd came in from the family gathering, mumbling to himself that there seemed to be a crisis every time he was on call during a special time such as a birthday, anniversary, or holiday.

"Mr. Cripps, we need to make a move," he said to the patient. "That blood is running out as fast as we can replace it."

"What if we wait?"

"Then you're in danger of bleeding to death."

Mr. Cripps acquiesced. The operation began at midnight and lasted three hours. A small section of duodenum containing the ulcer and the lower portion of the stomach, where most of the gastric acid is produced, were removed. The divided ends of stomach and duodenum were connected together. Then, the two vagus nerves at the top of the stomach were divided to divorce the mind from the stomach, since one phase of gastric acid secretion is stimulated by impulses from the brain.

Byrd stayed with Cripps in the recovery room until he felt satisfied that all was stable, and then he went home to bed and Santa. Two nights later he was awakened by his bedside telephone. It was Miss Hardacre, the night nurse. "I'm afraid Mr. Cripps is bleeding again, Doctor. He just passed a large, tarry black stool."

"How's his color?" he asked.

"It's ruddy," she replied.

"What about the pulse and blood pressure?"

"The pulses are 80 and the blood pressure is 140 over 78." For some reason, she characteristically referred to the pulse rate in the plural.

"Pretty normal," he said. "Well, Miss Hardacre, what you woke me for is to tell me good news, not bad. His intestine has been just lying there, all twenty feet of it, paralyzed by the insult of the surgery and full of blood from before surgery that hadn't passed through yet. Now, it's beginning to function again and move that old blood along. If it'll make you feel any better, get a hematocrit and hemoglobin." He was just getting back to sleep when the phone rang again.

"The blood counts are normal," she said.

This time Byrd couldn't get back to sleep, thinking how stupid he was not to tell her to call only if the blood level had dropped significantly.

The postoperative course progressed smoothly. Byrd and Cripps became good friends. A spiritual bond developed between them as a result of the life-threatening experience. In the course of conversation one day, Byrd asked, "What do you think your cows had to do with that ulcer, Cripps?"

"Well, you see, Dr. Byrd, I've been a dairy farmer for only the last five years. Before that I was a butler for a wealthy family in New York City."

"I had noticed that you don't talk like a Mainer," Byrd said.

"Actually, I was born in England. My parents

migrated to America when I was a small boy. My father was second cousin once removed of the Chancellor of the Exchequer in Britain, Sir Stafford Cripps. An idiotic BBC radio announcer once reported Sir Stafford's activities and mispronounced his name as Sir Stifford Crapps. Well, of course, the man was fired because of the blunder, but the damage was done. It was difficult for the family after that. Whenever our name was spoken, it brought an amused, knowing smile to the listener's face. Father was happy to begin a new life in a strange country where our name was unfamiliar."

Cripps continued, "My employers in New York were a very prominent family. They had a townhouse which I managed for them. They were sometimes away in Palm Beach or the south of France someplace. I was responsible for overseeing the work of the cook, the maid, and the chauffeur. I kept the pantry filled with all the best gourmet foods and the wine cellar well stocked, especially with Dom Perignon and their favorite Cabernet Sauvignon. There were frequent dinner parties to be planned, seating to be arranged, menus and floral arrangements to be looked after, house guests to be cared for. My employers were a cut above the rest, and that was the problem. I was a servant, a glorified slave so to speak, always at their beck and call. If everything wasn't arranged perfectly to their liking, it was my fault. I longed to be my own person, my own boss, not being told what to do at the whim of others. Also, I hated the dirty, noisy, crowded hectic city. I wanted to be free, live an idyllic life in the country, so I scrimped and saved. When the time came, I bought a dairy farm here in Maine from an elderly couple. I have a hundred acres of woods and pastures, a nice house, and a large barn."

"I gather it wasn't exactly what you expected," Byrd said.

"Hardly. First of all, my wife refused to leave the city. She divorced me. Our two sons, in their late teens, stayed with me. One liked the farm work, but the other didn't, so he later opened a 'Dairy Joy' near us and has a better income than his brother and I do put together. He even closes the place in the winter and goes to Florida."

"How many cattle do you have?" Byrd asked.

"Eighty-five milk cows, and then there are the calves, heifers, and bulls. What I didn't realize at the beginning is that you can never get a single day off. The cows have to be milked every day, twice, in fact. In the winter, which seems endless, you have to feed them, and in the summer when they're out in the pasture, you have to bring them all in for milking. The hay has to be mowed, baled, and stored in the barn. The manure has to be shoveled. The cows have to be assisted at calving time. Just try and hire a good herdsman. It's impossible. The good ones want their own farm, and the others are lazy, get drunk, and neglect the cows. I haven't had hardly a day off in five years. Not only that, but no matter how fastidious I am and how often I bathe, the odor of cow dung always lingers about my person. Wherever I go, people immediately know that I'm a dairy farmer, just from the stigma of that aroma. I am still a servant, but now it's changed to being a slave to cows instead of people. All they do is eat, chew their cud, drop turds all over the place, and stand there looking at me from under those long eyelashes."

"Well, Cripps, I think you're right," Byrd said.

"About what?" he asked.

"The cause of ulcers may not be known, but in your case, it is cows. Things should be better though, since we cut those nerves from your brain to your stomach. Stress can't stimulate your stomach to make acid."

Cripps went home to convalesce, then resume his life of servitude to his mistresses, the cows. Happily, however, everything eventually turned out the way he had dreamed. About five years later he returned to see Byrd at the office. He appeared tanned and fit. He walked in with an erect and dignified carriage, befitting his former occupation as a butler. A definite odor about him was evident and overpowering, but it wasn't cow dung. Byrd recognized it as Brut aftershave lotion. Cripps was attired as usual in black clothes. No doubt he must be a Johnny Cash fan, Byrd thought. Cripps rolled his black t-shirt up and pulled his black shorts down to display a bulging hernia in the left groin.

"I've ruptured myself," he said.

"Any idea how that happened?"

"I sold the land to a condominium developer for a handsome profit, sold off all the cattle, married a fine widow, and just work around the house now. I've fixed up the farm pond with a fountain in the middle. A bunch of ducks swim around in it. I've put a couple of plastic, pink flamingoes in the edge to dress it up a bit."

"What's that got to do with the hernia?"

"Well, I'm building a rock garden on the slope next to the house. That's how I got the rupture, lifting all those rocks."

Byrd was relieved that the ulcer problem had not recurred, and that the source of it had been removed. It was a relatively simple project to repair the hernia. J. Hartwell Cripps went home from the hospital with a promise not to lift any more rocks for six weeks. At last he was a free man.

The Harbor Master

Athelbert Church was a craggy-faced fisherman well over six feet tall and a bit on the portly side. His lower lip, to which a cigarette was usually attached, protruded over his square jaw, giving him a rather belligerent appearance. The muscles of the lids under his blue eyes had given up after long years of squinting against the sun, rain, and wind. The eyelids hung down to expose their red lining. Beneath each lower lid was an edematous pouch. A person looking at Bert was reminded of a sad-eyed hound dog except that his large ears didn't hang down.

Except for the time during the war when he was in the Coast Guard, Bert lived all his life on Partridge Neck. By the time he reached his seventieth year, he was so used up with arthritis that he couldn't haul lobster traps anymore, but he kept his high prowed, beamy, thirty-two-foot Nova Scotia fishing boat. He loved the way that old boat hunkered down and cut through rough seas with hardly a degree of pitch or roll. The summer people hired Bert to take their children out on the bay to fish or just to look at the scenery. Sometimes, he took the children over to Bar Harbor and tied up at the dock and waited while the children ran whooping and laughing into town to buy ice cream cones. When the occasion presented itself, Bert would go out in his boat and pull alongside a sardine carrier while it was sucking up thrashing and wriggling fish from a purse seine into its hold with a big vacuum hose. He would trade a few bottles of orange soda for the mackerel that the crew separated out from the sardines and didn't want anyway.

Most of the time in the summer Bert just sat on the shore or in his old pickup truck next to the dock, looking out across the bay past the boats riding at their moorings. Early in the morning he'd watch the sun come up behind Schoodic Mountain. After dark, the truck was still there, and you could tell by the red glow of a cigarette behind the steering wheel that Bert was in it. In fact, he sat at the dock so much that the town fathers appointed him harbor master, a position which they never saw the need for previously, and for which they could pay him a pittance. His duties were to assign cruising yachts to the guest moorings and keep the young sports in their motor boats from kicking up too much of a wake in the harbor. The heavy work, such as setting the big granite moorings and periodically changing their heavy chains when they rusted, was done by a young man from across the bay who owned a big rugged boat. There wasn't much of a harbor anyway, just a shallow concavity along the east shore of the peninsula. Autumn and winter storms roared in past the islands that ringed the bay, and every few years the dock was smashed off its granite footings. The summer people always had it rebuilt before the next sailing season.

Bert lived in a snug, sparsely furnished, square, little house nestled in the pine and spruce trees at the foot of a hill, well back from the waterfront. In his opinion houses built by the sea were damp and took too much of a beating from the salt spray and wind to be practical. It was preferable to let the visitors from New Jersey and Pennsylvania stay on the water's edge in the summer and pay for the oft-needed repairs, not to mention the higher town taxes.

For several years Bert had been happily married to a sweet woman who gave piano lessons to the town children, but she had died young and left him without offspring. Bert's needs were few, since he raised most of what he ate, and he heated the house with wood that he cut in the forest. He tended his vegetable garden behind the house. Some chickens were in the dooryard, and racks of splayed out salt cod and pollock hung drying in the sun. Jars of vegetables, pickles, boysenberry, and strawberry jam lined the shelves in tidy rows down under in the cool, granite-lined cellar of the house. Sacks of potatoes, squash, dried beans for baking, onions, and turnips sat on wooden frames just above the dirt floor. So, Bert's material needs were clearly not great, and he was quite content to live frugally. He had his home, his boat, and plenty of food.

Once, a real estate man had tried to sell him a small island not far offshore in the bay for $5,000. Bert went slowly around the island on the water, observing its bold shore and rocky cliffs crowned by spruce and fir trees. Then he went ashore on a small pebbly beach at the foot of a green meadow and walked all over the island. Next time he saw the salesman, Bert said, "She's a beauty, all right, but what would I do with an island?"

Ten years later the real estate agent told Bert, "That island was just resold for $40,000. You could have made a killing if you'd bought it when you had the chance."

Bert looked at him for a minute and then replied. "What would I do with $40,000?"

One day Bert bumped into Myrtice Pettengill outside the village store where Bert had gone to buy a carton of unfiltered Camels and some aspirin for his arthritis. They had known each other since grammar school. She was a slim, wiry, neatly dressed woman with gray hair pulled back in a bun. Myrtice had been married to Ivory Pettengill for fifty years. They had three children, all grown and moved away with their own families. She had worked long and hard years in the woods with her woodcutter husband. On this particular day Myrtice was in what could be called a high dudgeon.

"Bert, I've had it up to here with Ivory," she said, indicating her upper neck in front. "He's always been mean and miserable, but since he retired, it's just getting worse and worse. All he does is sit there in the overstuffed chair, stare at the TV set, drink beer, belch, and break wind. Once in awhile he'll scratch his old rabbit hound's ears when he isn't scratching himself. And you know that grey color he has. There's not a thing wrong with his heart or his blood. It's just plain dirt. I swear the last time that man took a bath was when his mother's water broke."

"Well, I never thought Ivory was such a bad old feller, Myrtice, even if his eyes are too close together. You can't trust a man whose eyes are too close together, or for that matter a bilateral combacross either."

"What's a bilateral combacross?" she asked.

"You don't know? Why that's a man who's bald on top, lets the side fringes grow long, and combs them across, one side to the other to cover up the bald part. A man like that will always try to cover up his mistakes, even though it's not his fault that his hair fell out."

"Ivory's bald enough, but he's never done that. I wouldn't want to put the idea in his mind though. I'm leaving him after fifty years. It's final. Enough's enough."

"Myrtice, if you're so bound and determined to leave Ivory, you could just move in with me," Bert said.

So she did. And they got along quite well together. The fires of passion had long since been banked for both of them, of course. Ivory didn't seem to mind the transfer. In fact, he seemed almost pleased to be rid of her. She kept Bert's house neat and clean, mended his shirts, and darned his socks. They rode around together in the old pickup, parked down by the dock, and even went to the annual square dance at the village green on a warm summer night. Of course, they just sat in the pickup, listening to the music, and watching from the darkness beyond the fringe of laughing and prancing dancers of all ages. The only thing that anyone could see inside the cab of the truck was the red glow of Bert's cigarette. There was an elbow sticking out of the open cab window on each side, his brown and hers white.

163

One summer Harry Byrd decided to rent a cottage on Partridge Neck to get his wife and children away from the city. His vacation was only for two weeks, but it was in the best part of the summer, straddling the end of July and the first part of August. He joined his family on alternate weekends when he was off call. One hot sunny day Harry walked his children down to the dock to go swimming and give their mother some peace and quiet for awhile. That's when he met Athelbert Church, who was sitting on a rock in the shade under an old apple tree a few yards above the line of seaweed that formed the high water mark. They watched the children running in and out of the frigid ocean water, jumping off the dock, and laughing and screaming in delight.

"Look at them," Bert said. "They're in the prime of life and don't even know it. If you or I did that, we'd turn all blue and probably have a heart attack."

"Is that cold water why most lobster fisherman never learn to swim?" Harry asked.

"Well, I learned to swim over at the old abandoned granite quarry, but a man can't last long in this water if his boat goes down, even in the summer and even if he could swim," Bert said.

"That's quite a view you have here with those mountains rising out of the sea across the bay," Harry said.

"Yep, that's the highest point of land on the east coast from here to Rio de Janeiro. We say here in Partridge Neck that those people across there in Bar Harbor at the foot of the mountains are sitting on their own view."

The next Sunday morning the Byrd family stopped

by the dock on their way home from church services to admire the view. Athelbert Church was sitting under the apple tree.

"Why are you people all dressed up like that?" he asked.

"We're just on our way back from church," Harry said.

"Hah! Church is for hypocrites. This is my church right here. There's no better place to worship the Lord and praise his works," Bert said.

"Why do you say hypocrites, Bert?"

"Because I know those mealy-mouthed, sancti-monious psalm singers. They go to church on Sunday, then all the rest of the week they go right back to lying, meanness, slander, and malicious cheating. The last time I went to church was for the funeral of one of my friends. He was an old reprobate, and everybody knew it. I knew his faults, and he knew mine, but I didn't hold it against him. I liked him just the same. That's what a friend is. When the minister got through with his preaching and praising the dear departed one, I didn't have any idea who in hell he was talking about. Certainly, it couldn't have been my lazy, fat friend who drank too much, never did a whole day's work in his life, and tried to play grab ass with all the women. The pews were groaning from the weight of a bunch of women all blowing their noses and dabbing their eyes with hankies. I swore, right then and there, never to go into a church again."

"Come on now, Bert. You shouldn't tar all people who go to church with the same brush," Harry said.

"Maybe not, but there are a lot of them, that's for sure," Bert replied.

Whenever Harry went down to the dock, he chatted with Bert, and gradually the two became friends, even though the old fisherman regarded most summer people with disdain. Harry felt a certain kinship with him in that regard because as a summer renter, his family was not accepted by the cottage owners who had summered at Partridge Neck for multiple generations. Harry and Avis were never invited to their frequent cocktail parties or their evening discussions of the great books, which was fine with him, but when he passed by any of them while walking along the shore road, and Harry smiled in his usual friendly fashion, he was answered with cold, blank stares. He might as well have been an invisible man. Athelbert Church understood this, although it puzzled Harry Byrd.

"You will never be accepted here by those people, Harry," he said. "If your family keeps coming back though, your grandchildren might be. Most of the owners are teachers, musicians, writers, college professors, or ministers, who have inherited their cottages from their forebears. Partridge Neck summer people are long on brains and short on money. Of course, over in Blue Hill it's the other way around. We natives are treated the same way you are. They use us to mow their lawns, saw up their trees that blow over in storms, and keep an eye on their property in the winter, but they consider themselves a cut above us." Byrd decided that was a pretty good explanation of the relationship between the summer people and the rest of the world.

As the two walked over toward the dock, Harry

noted Bert walked quite stiffly. Bert complained, "When I get up in the morning, every joint is stiff."

"Have you seen a rheumatologist about it?" Byrd asked.

"I did once, and he gave me gold injections. Lot of good that did. I would have been better off with the gold in my pocket instead of under the hide. It's not as bad in the summer as it gets in the winter, though."

"Maybe it would help if you could go someplace warm like Florida or Arizona in the winter," Byrd said.

"A few winters back before Myrtice moved in, my nephew, Basil Ellingwood, and his wife Ella took me along with them down to Florida in their big Winnebago. Seemed like we drove forever to get there, and the next day I was ready to come home. Too many old people down there all driving around in big cars and jamming up the roads. Some of them even have bumper stickers saying 'I'm spending my children's inheritance.' You have to stand in line for everything at the restaurants, the supermarket, the laundromat, and even at the post office just to buy stamps. The same tourists you see over at Bar Harbor in the summer are down there in the winter, or at least they look the same. They wear loud colored shorts, dark sunglasses with a ribbon around the neck so they won't lose the glasses, black socks, and a T-shirt reading 'I heart New York'. They all have big pot bellies, hairy legs, and knobby knees. Everyone of them has a camera around his neck, radio earphones with an antenna sticking up like some kind of big weird bug, and a poodle on a leash. The young people down there who work seem to be providing services for the old people, and a lot of the young folks don't work at all. They just lie on the beach drinking beer and popping these pills called Quaaludes. Then there are all kinds of retirement facilities with names like 'Century Center'. Just that name lures the old folks in. The idea is that if they stay there, they'll live to be a hundred. We went to a supermarket across the street from one of those places, and it was full of old ladies tearing around the aisles with their shopping carts, glaring at anyone who dared to get in their way. Their poor, pussy-whipped husbands trailed behind, as if each of them was on a chain with a nose ring. You risk your life walking around in a store like that. In fact, I found out from one of the clerks there that one of the old ladies nearly killed the store manager."

"Now come on, Bert. How could that be?" Harry asked.

"Well, he was putting some Wheaties boxes back on the shelf after an old lady knocked them over. Another old lady came tearing along and whacked him in the back of his ankle with her shopping cart. She ruptured his heel cord," Bert said.

"That certainly would put him out of commission for a few weeks, but it wouldn't be life-threatening," Harry said.

"Just hold on a damned minute. I'm coming to that," Bert said. "The manager developed a blood clot in the leg. It traveled and hit him in the lung. He ended up in the intensive care unit but recovered eventually. If I were that supermarket manager, I'd get myself and everyone in the store crew, except the girls at the checkout counter where they are protected, a set of those hockey shin guards and have everybody wear them on the back of their legs instead of the front."

"Was there anything about Florida that you liked Bert?" Harry asked.

"There was one thing, and that was the zoo. It wasn't like your ordinary zoo. Instead of the animals being kept in cages, the people were in cages. Everybody had to stay inside their automobiles and drive along the winding dirt roads in the zoo to watch the animals and birds all roaming around free in this big area of fields, trees, and ponds. The zoo keepers kept them all well fed, so they didn't attack each other. Young men drove around in zebra-striped pickup trucks to tend the animals and make sure the people didn't get out of their cars. I made one mistake, though. It was a hot day, so I had a couple of beers while we were driving out to the zoo. By the time we finished looking and driving around all those winding roads, my bladder was about to burst. You don't buy beer you know, you just rent it. I couldn't get out to take a leak until we got to the refreshment area at the end. If I'd had my wits about me, there would have been an empty coffee can in the car for relief."

"It was worth it, though. There was an elephant eating oranges and some vegetables on the ground. A peacock came sneaking up between his legs and tried to steal some of his food. I never thought I'd see an elephant chasing a peacock. Of course, that big awkward critter never could catch him. The peacock scampered around, staying just out of reach. Then we saw a baby rhinoceros playing games with his mother. He'd run full tilt at her on his little stumpy legs and bang head on into her ribs from the side. The old lady just looked around at him, slightly annoyed. Good thing he hadn't grown the horn on the front of his forehead yet or she might have had to teach him a lesson. We saw monkeys swinging around in the trees, and two spindly giraffes walked across the road right in front of us. The lions weren't all that ferocious. The ones we saw were all asleep on their backs with their feet sticking up in the air. The ostriches were something else, though. Those crazy-looking giant birds have long skinny legs with feet that look too big for them. Their bodies are about the size and shape of a lobster trap with feathers. Sticking up from the top, they have this neck that's even longer and skinnier than their legs. On top of that they have a dumb-looking face with a few spears of feathers standing straight up on a bald pink head. We saw this one particular ostrich prancing up and down in circles around another ostrich that was lying on the ground beating its short, stubby, useless-looking wings on the dirt and jerking its bald head around like a tennis ball on the end of a pole. It must have been a mating dance because the next thing we knew the dancing ostrich hopped on top of the one on the ground. Ella was so embarrassed that she had to turn her face away and look out the other window at the trees. Me and Basil felt like a couple of them voyeurs, so we drove off to see the rest of the sights."

"The only things at the zoo that they kept in cages were the snakes–water moccasins, copperheads, and coral snakes. It's a good thing we don't have any of those ugly, poisonous critters in Maine. They'd freeze to death in the winter, although those harmless little garter snakes seem to survive all right. The snakes were at the refreshment area outside the fence of the zoo. There were flower gardens there and a dirt track for elephant rides. The kids climbed up a set of stairs to a platform and stepped into a big box with seats on the elephant's back. Then a trainer in white pants and shirt, carrying a boat hook, led him around the track. While we were watching, another elephant was brought in to relieve the working one who was then washed down with a hose and a push broom. Next thing you know the man in the trainer suit brought up a regular galvanized trash barrel and held it under the elephant's hind end. The elephant promptly obliged him and just about filled that barrel. The trainer could barely carry it off, it was so full. I never thought I'd see a housebroken elephant, but there it was, bigger than life and twice as ugly!"

"How were your joints in that warm winter climate, Bert?" Harry asked.

"Not a bit different," Bert said. "I'd never go back there again. It's not worth traveling 1500 miles each way just to go to a zoo. You might say it's a long run for a short slide. When we drove over the Piscataqua River on that new bridge from New Hampshire into Maine, I was so happy that all my toes curled up. I had to open the window and take a big gulp of cold, clear Maine air. The way I look at it, the falling snow cleans and filters the air. Not only that, but it keeps the germs down so they can't blow around in the dust like they do down south. That clean white snow on the ground and on the trees is beautiful to look at as long as I don't have to work in the woods or go out on the water any more."

One day Bert said to Harry, "You know, you're the

only bootcher I know except for Dick Taylor at the Shop & Save supermarket in Ellsworth. Maybe sometime I could come up to see you about this rupture I got from hauling traps a few years back."

"I noticed you have a bulge in your pants and figured it was either that or you were overly endowed," Harry said.

Athelbert Church, accompanied by Myrtice Pettengill, appeared for an appointment at Harry Byrd's office during the spring of the next year. "Myrtice here has a problem she wants to talk to you about," Bert said. "If you can get her fixed up, I'll take care of her afterwards, then you can fix my rupture, and she'll take care of me."

"What's the problem?" Harry asked.

Myrtice answered, "Back when I was working in the woods with Ivory, I pulled on a Peavey to turn a log and hove my womb right inside out. When I'm standing up, it hangs out, and when I lie down, it goes back up inside."

"How come you waited so long to get it fixed?" Byrd asked.

"Well, it really didn't bother me all that much, but lately it hangs half way down to my knees and drags on my bladder. I have to pee every half hour or so during the day. I'm all right at night when I push it back up inside where it belongs."

"Do you have any other health problems or have you had any injuries?"

"No injuries, although I did fall twenty feet off a ladder one time when I was painting the house."

"Did you break anything?"

"Just my grape arbor. I've never been sick in my life,

just had the three babies. All big ones, they were, ten pounders. That stretched me up pretty good down below, and then hauling logs all those years didn't help any."

"I believe you're probably right, Myrtice," Byrd said. "That certainly could do it."

An examination confirmed the obvious. She, indeed, had a prolapsed uterus. Hospital arrangements were made, and Myrtice underwent a vaginal hysterectomy and repair of the damaged supporting muscles in her pelvis to hold the urinary bladder in its proper position. She made a smooth postoperative recovery and walked out of the hospital, announcing to her nurse that she felt like a spring chicken.

Six weeks later Bert and Myrtice returned to see Byrd at his office. She had recovered her energy, and the examination showed that she had healed well.

"I'm ready to get this damned rupture fixed now," Bert said.

"How's your health, otherwise?" Bert asked.

"Fine, except for the arthritis. Maybe while you're at it, you could squirt some WD-40 into my joints. The knees, elbows, hips, and back are all stiff and creaky."

"Now besides hauling lobster traps, other kinds of straining can cause a hernia, like straining from bowel problems for instance, or difficulty in urination from prostate gland enlargement. Coughing can do it, too," Harry said.

"My vent works fine, and there's no problem with the waterworks. I do have some cough, though. Every morning I have to clear out the tubes."

"Sometimes, it's so bad I think he's going to cough up his shoes," Myrtice added.

"How much do you smoke?" Harry asked.

"Around four packs a day, and don't go telling me how bad that is. My friend, Eben Spurling, over on Cranberry Island smoked as much as I do, or more, and he lived to be a hundred. When he was eighty, he sold his house and land to a couple from Philadelphia to use for a summer place. The contract was that they paid him the whole price, but he could stay right there 'til he died. Then they would take everything over. Eben outlived them both as it turned out. You might say he outslickered the city slickers, and neither one of them ever smoked. Personally, I think he lived that long on account of what he ate."

"What was special about his diet?" Byrd asked.

"It was porridge. A couple of times a day he ate a bowl of cornmeal, chopped up potato, and salt codfish, all mixed in together with some milk and heated up on the stove. Of course, in the summer he had a garden and ate plenty of fresh vegetables out of it."

"Now, Bert, you know that doesn't prove a thing about smoking, except that Eben was one of the lucky ones. It sounds like his diet was low in fat, and he probably had good genes," Byrd said.

"Yes, that's true. All his forebears were long lived. I suppose you're right about the smoking, Harry, but it's too late for me to stop now after sixty years."

The two went into the adjacent examining room. Bert took off his green twill shirt and trousers. Underneath he wore a one piece suit of clean white drawers with buttons down the front and a vertical single buttoned split in the tail. It covered him from wrists to ankles. "When do you change over to summer underwear, Bert? Here it is July, and you're still wearing long drawers," Harry said.

"This is my summer underwear. In the winter I wear a much heavier union suit. I keep out the winter cold and the summer heat," Bert said.

The hernia was a giant one, with half of Bert's intestines lying in the big protrusion that extended down from his right groin into the greatly distended scrotum. "We can stuff everything back inside your abdomen where it belongs and repair the defect in your groin muscles all right, Bert. It might also just help to keep the hernia from recurring, since it's so large, if we take out the testicle on that side. The cord to the testicle makes a weak place where it comes through the groin from inside."

"Well, I don't know about that. Maybe we should see what Myrtice thinks about it," Bert said.

He dressed and they went back to the office where she was waiting. "Dr. Byrd here says it would be a good idea to take out the stone on that right side to help shove things up when he fixes the rupture. What do you think about that, Myrtice?"

"I'm against it," she said.

"It wouldn't make him any less of a man, Myrtice. One testicle is just as good as two," Byrd said. "He wouldn't be castrated like one of those eunuchs."

"That may be, but I like it the way it is. It makes him look so dressy," she said.

"That settles it," Bert said.

"All right, we'll leave it in," Harry said. "And oh, one other thing. I noticed you have all those little white scars on the front of your chest. What caused them?"

"Those are caused by my arthritis."

"What?"

"It's like this. The joint pains wake me up at night, so I take a couple of aspirin and have a smoke while I wait for the pain to quiet down," Bert said.

"Yes, and then he falls asleep smoking. He burns the front of him right through his nightshirt," Myrtice said. "One night he came running down the stairs with the smouldering mattress over his head. He went right past me while I was knitting in the rocking chair and threw the mattress out the door into the snow in the dooryard. After that, I made him keep a bucket of water beside the bed next to his chamber pot."

"Fat lot of good that did," Bert said. "I woke up from the burning and emptied the bucket on my chest, but all I got was a bruise because it's so cold in my room that the water had froze stiff."

"Now, that's a new twist on the evils of smoking," Byrd said.

The following week Harry Byrd repaired the hernia and pushed all those loops of bowel back inside Bert's abdomen where they belonged, even though they had lost the right of eminent domain. Bert recovered rapidly. His main complaint was that his belly was bigger, and he had to let his belt out a couple of notches. At the time of Bert's discharge from the hospital, Byrd strongly admonished him not to lift anything heavy or pull on the oars of his dinghy for six weeks.

It wasn't long before Bert was back at the dock,

sitting in his pickup or under the apple tree, looking at the view. He lived to be eighty-seven years old. Of course, smoking shortened his life. Otherwise, he probably would have lived to be a hundred. He might have observed, "Who wants to live to be a hundred like those people at the Century Center down in Florida."

Missing

The two Hawkes brothers took two weeks off every spring right after Memorial Day and went fishing. Wilbur, a pediatrician, was in his late forties and Wesley, an obstetrician, was ten years his senior. Unlike most people who angle for trout and landlocked salmon on the many lakes and ponds of Piscataquis County, they preferred brook fishing. It was too boring for them to sit in a boat on a lake all day. They owned an old cabin that was nestled in the white birch and tall pines on the shore of Roach Pond, just east of Moosehead Lake. Each day they rose at sunup and ate a good breakfast. Then they packed a lunch and set out with their light fishing gear along the Pleasant River, which flows through the valley between Whitecap and Big Shanty Mountains on one side and Chairback and Baker Mountains on the other. All day they followed the streams and brooks that tumble down the slopes of the mountains. The swollen streams rushed in the spring from the melting snow. Periodically, the brothers cast a fly from the shore or waded into the water to cast into a tempting pool. The dense, fragrant forest rose like a green wall on all sides and surrounded the fishermen. The silence was interrupted by the soft rustle of wind in the trees, the birds singing to each other, and the soothing sound of water flowing over and around the rocks in the stream bed. Occasionally, deer and moose came cautiously out of the forest to drink from the stream. In late afternoon Wilbur and Wesley cleaned their catch of brook trout and returned to camp, physically tired but mentally refreshed. When two weeks had passed, the burdens of the long winter and the stresses of their lives were washed away, renewing them in body and spirit. Their wives didn't seem to resent the annual spousal absence. Perhaps, it made them easier to live with, although, like most fishermen, they were gentle people.

One bright June morning word came to town that one of the Hawkes brothers had disappeared in the woods. They had set out on the previous day along the west branch of the Pleasant River, one going upstream and the other downstream. The plan was for them to meet in the late afternoon. At the appointed time, Wes didn't appear, so Wil waited. His anxiety slowly increased. He searched down along the stream and found no sign of his brother. He went back to seek help from the game warden, but that took more time and dusk was falling. A search party couldn't hope to accomplish anything at night in the forest.

When Harry Byrd came out of the operating room that morning after completing a gallbladder removal, he was told that Wesley Hawkes was missing in the North Woods, and the news hit him like a physical blow. Both brothers were his friends, but Wilbur was a special person. He had saved two of Byrd's newborn children from brain damage, or more likely death, by doing exchange transfusions because of RH factor blood incompatibility. In those days, it was necessary to spend hours suctioning the infant's self-destructing blood through the umbilical vein and replacing it with new compatible blood, two ounces out, two ounces in until all the newborn's original blood had been exchanged. Byrd had often observed Wil pacing in the physicians' lounge at the hospital with furrowed brow and worried eyes because a child or infant under his care was not doing well. Wil couldn't rest easily until that child was out of danger. Now, Byrd could see him, distraught and sleepless, waiting for dawn so the search for his brother could begin.

It was clear to Byrd that he had to go and help in the search. He arranged with a surgeon friend to look after his patients, and he went to a woodsmen's outfitting store for some heavy boots, green wool trousers, and a red and black plaid jacket, thick enough to keep out the cold and blackflies.

"I'm going up to Piscataquis County and help look for Wesley Hawkes," he announced to his wife.

"You're out of your mind, Harry. You know you've been lost in the supermarket. What help would you be in the woods? We don't need two lost people," Avis said.

Byrd looked hurt. "I wasn't lost in the supermarket. It just took a long time to find all those things on your shopping list, like Bing cherries and Mandarin oranges. Those Pillsbury breadsticks turned out to be in the dairy section for some reason, not to mention the cheeze dip that wasn't in the cracker section but with potato chips. Besides,

I'm going with Bob Goslin."

Avis reluctantly agreed once he mentioned Bob Goslin, a surgeon friend of theirs. Everyone called him "Goose," of course. He'd been born and raised in Aroostook County and was an accomplished fisherman, hunter, and a lover of the outdoors. He had manned a firewatch tower on a mountain in the forest during the summer while he was a student at the University of Maine. It didn't have anything to do with his part-time occupation, but Goslin was built sort of like a fire hydrant.

"All right, go. I haven't forgotten what Wil did for us when we needed him," she said.

So, Harry Byrd and Goose Goslin drove up to Moosehead Lake, went along its east shore, then turned off onto the bumpy, rutted, dirt road at Kokadjo. After about four hours, they arrived at the search area before nightfall. There they found many men, including game wardens, volunteer woodsmen, fishermen, friends, and family of the missing man.

A smiling lady served hot coffee and sandwiches out of the back of a Red Cross van. Periodically, float planes from Greenville flew low overhead, searching from the air. The wardens had organized the men into groups of ten each and had a systematic plan to search along the Pleasant River and its branches, Bear Brook, White Brook, Gulf Hagas Brook, East Chairback Brook, and others. No sign of Wesley Hawkes had been found on the first day, and there was much more territory to cover.

Byrd and Goslin were assigned for the night to one of the log cabins at a sporting camp on West Branch Pond.

Eight small log cabins and a larger central one were scattered along the shore of the pond, each with its own outhouse in back. Directly across, on the other side of the lake, rose White Cap Mountain with a big green scar across its face where the trees had been clear cut many years before. The log cabins were simply furnished with two beds, two chairs, a pine table, and a potbellied woodstove. A single, bare light bulb hung from the ceiling for use until 9:00pm when the camp electric generator was shut off for the night. Wood for the stove was stacked on the front porch. Harry built a fire in the stove while Goose broke out the bottle of Canadian whisky which he had the foresight to bring along. They each had half a tumblerful to warm their insides while the fire warmed their surface. Then they walked over to one of the other cabins to visit Wilbur and Marian, Wesley's wife. She was distraught and fretting, just as they expected, and she was pretty hyper, making all sorts of plans for the next day with her two sons.

"One of Wesley's patients called me on the phone," she said. "Wes had come to her in a dream last night and said he was next to a big, black rock. I know it's probably foolish, but we've got to go looking for big, black rocks tomorrow. I've even hired a psychic to come up and help us, for whatever good that might do."

"Worry does funny things to people," Byrd said softly to Goslin, who nodded in sympathetic agreement.

Next morning they were up at first light. While they ate breakfast in the main cabin, they watched the big, orange sun come up in the clear blue sky above the lake. They greeted Joe Merganser, an orthopedic surgeon from town, and Trudy, his wife, who were sitting at a nearby table.

"Great morning. You both come up to look for Wesley?" Goose asked.

"No, we come up here every spring to fish," Joe said. "This is our favorite place."

Byrd was sort of disgusted. "How the hell can they sit out on the lake all day fishing with Wes lost in the woods someplace?" he quietly said to Goslin.

"Different people just have different ideas about what's important, I guess," Goose replied.

Harry thought about that a couple of years later when Joe Merganser died of a brain tumor at age 53 and wished he hadn't thought ill of him for fishing at the wrong time, since he never did get many more chances to fish. The first malignant cells might well have been starting to germinate back then.

As they were leaving to join the search party, Pat Dow, who owned the camps and whose father-in-law had built them, was pointing out the best fishing locations on the lake to a sporting type from New Jersey or someplace. The greenhorn was nattily attired in his Abercrombie and Fitch togs with outside pockets all over the jacket, a creel to put his fish in, and trout flies stuck all around the band of his Australian-style felt hat with the brim turned up on one side.

"Right over by that big dead pine is good," Pat said, "and I've taken many a trout in the big cove at the other end of the lake. Right across where you see that old bull moose with his head underwater eating grass is excellent fishing, too. Don't worry about the moose attacking you. They only get mean in the rutting season which isn't 'til fall."

The screen door slammed shut on its spring just behind the sport as he hurried down to the line of rowboats at the dock. Pat's hoarse bellow followed him out. "Of course, we don't guarantee nuthin."

Many times in later years Byrd remembered that admonition and felt like saying the same to patients before taking them to the operating room for a serious problem. Nowadays, if a surgeon doesn't get a perfect result, he may find himself sitting in a courtroom.

The game warden in charge of the search was Henri Jalbert, known to everybody as "Hank." There was bad blood between him and Goslin, who had sworn to castrate Hank if he ever had the opportunity. He actually did have the opportunity once, but passed it up. When Hank was in the hospital to have his shoulder separation repaired, the orthopedic surgeon called Goose the night before surgery.

"Jalbert will be asleep while I fix his shoulder in the morning. Here's the chance you've been looking for."

Goose explained. "One time I was fishing from the dam on Moosehead Lake at the east outlet of the Kennebec River. I knew the Fish and Game Department rules prohibited fishing on the outlet side of the dam. I heard this splash behind me in the outlet, turned around, and cast the fly into the ripples where the fish had risen. Hank rose right up out of the bushes and put the arm on me. I got a hundred dollar fine later at the County Seat in Dover-Foxcroft. The more I thought about it, the more I was sure that splash wasn't a fish after all, but a stone tossed by old Hank just to trap me."

"Why would he do that?" Byrd asked.

"Don't know, unless he was still mad because one time the judge let me off. I got off when Hank accused me of blasting away at some honking Canada geese flying over the camp at night. The only evidence he had was a bunch of feathers, and I claimed I was shooting at a fox that was pestering the camp."

In any event Hank assigned Goslin and Byrd to the worst job, which was to sweep with a group of other men through the woods along the Pleasant River. The men were about fifty feet apart in a line. Goose was on Byrd's left, and on his right was a slim, leathery, old woodsman who looked to be in his sixties. He didn't talk at all, and he emanated a powerful odor, like a combination of skunk and garlic, which Goslin explained was due to asafetida to repel the blackflies. Goose had an endless store of useless knowledge.

"Asafetida is a gum resin that comes from a plant grown in Afghanistan. It's been used as a laxative, expectorant, sedative, and in France they use it as a condiment, greatly diluted, of course. Those Frenchmen will eat anything, even eels, and snails, which aren't anything but slugs in a shell. This particular fly dope has never been popular because it repels everything, including people, which is all right with that old woodsman because he doesn't have much use for people, anyway."

The black flies in the woods swarmed around Byrd, who covered every inch of his skin that he could. The woodsman was untouched by the cloud of insects around him because of his invisible wall of repellant. Byrd went stumbling along through the dense forest, whipped by evergreen branches. He kept tripping when his new boots caught in projecting roots that looked like miniature McDonald's golden arches. Goose Goslin was managing quite well on his left, and on the right the old woodsman went gliding along through the woods as if he were walking down Main Street. From time to time, he'd wait for the others to catch up.

All that Harry Byrd found that day was a porcupine eating the bark off a doomed, young pine tree and a family of partridges that suddenly took off right in front of him with a great noisy thrashing of wings that startled Byrd. At first he was afraid that he might have stumbled on a bear with such a racket. There was no sign of the missing man, not unexpectedly, for why should he be in the deep forest unless he had lost his mind, which was unlikely. The men who had the easier job of searching along the streams had no better luck, as they found out when all returned to the base camp before sundown.

That evening Byrd and Goslin utilized a generous amount of the Canadian whisky again and were pretty relaxed when they went over to the main cabin for dinner. The roast beef, mashed potatoes, canned string beans, apple pie, and coffee tasted especially good after thrashing around in the woods all day. Joe Merganser even shared some of his fresh caught, pink-fleshed, broiled trout with them.

Back at the cabin they turned in early before the electric generator was shut off, but first they stood out on the porch awhile, leaning on the railing. It was cold, clear, windless moonlit night. The lake was black and smooth except for intermittent widening ripples, each preceded by the faint splash of a trout rising for an insect on the surface.

The shadows of symmetrical pointed fir and jagged irregular pines along the opposite shore were dark and forbidding. The night sky was filled with so many more stars than Byrd was used to seeing in the city. Goslin had studied the constellations during his summers on the fire tower.

"There's Polaris, the North Star," he said. "That's Draco, the Dragon and Casseiopeia's Chair, shaped like a "W", Ursa Major and Minor, the Big and Little Dippers, you know, anyway. I once knew a sea captain who looked at those stars so much that he named his son, Orion."

Every five minutes a siren wailed in the distance. "What the wardens do is place a lighted, portable siren up on the hill on each side of the valley. A lost person can go to the sound, read the instructions on the siren, and turn it off, marking his location to the rescuers," Goslin said.

The only other sound in the night was the eerie call of the loons on the lake. Goslin again reached into his store of fascinating information. "Loons have five separate and distinct calls," he said. "One is for staking out territory, another for letting each other know their location. A third call is to signal alarm, and the fourth is the mating call. I can't remember what the fifth call is, but I figure that on a lovely June night like this, we're listening to loon love songs."

They slept well that night after the exertion of the day and the good Canadian whisky. Next morning the skies were leaden, and a cold drizzle lasted all day. This time, in another sector of the woods, Byrd was a little better adjusted to the task and managed to avoid the whipping branches and most of the golden arches. That afternoon Wesley Hawkes was found. Warden Hank Jalbert had gone back along Bear Brook on a hunch, even though he had been there the day before. He turned off along a small side branch of the brook, and after a few yards there was Wesley, hidden by the dense foliage. His fishing rod stood upright against a tree, and next to it, Wesley had been cleaning his fish, with his feet in the water. He had just toppled over right there, peaceful as can be, apparently taken by a heart attack. It was a good way to go for Wesley, but mighty hard on his family and everybody else.

Later, Byrd and Goslin paid their condolences to Wil, Marian, and her sons. They packed their few things for the trip back. There wasn't much Canadian whisky left in the bottle, so they left it on the table.

"How much do we owe you for the meals and lodging, Pat?" Harry asked.

"Nuthin," replied their host. "Considerin' why you come up here, not exactly for fun. Be glad to have you back another time to fish, and I'll charge you for that."

Avis was relieved when Harry got back to town, and she never worried again about sending him to the supermarket, where, of course, he was not exactly anxious to go.

Byrd did take up Pat Down's invitation and took Avis as well as their five children up to the lake. The boys learned fly fishing and caught enough trout to keep them happy. The youngest child was more interested in the bloodsuckers attached to the fish entrails in the water where the trout had been cleaned. Avis and Harry fished, too, but the beauty of the area was enough for them just by itself. They went back to Piscataquis County every spring for many years, but they never did try brook fishing.

The Ancient One

Everybody loved Effie Haskell, not only because of her steadfast love of friend and neighbor, but also because of her cheerful disposition and proven durability. She was a ninety-three-year-old widow who lived alone in the home that her husband, Asa, had built in Eastport, Maine, where they had both spent their entire lives. He ran a boatyard and had died in his sixties of what Effie referred to as a "bum ticker." Their son and only child took over the operation of the boatyard when his father became disabled.

Effie's house was a small, white clapboard, center-chimney Cape that looked out on the sea and the rocky, fir-clad offshore islands. Inside, the house was neatly kept and immaculately clean. The furnishings were an antique dealer's dream, but Effie wasn't about to sell them off because of the memories they held for her. She was in good health except for some rheumatism, which didn't slow her down much. Her father had taught her that it is better to wear out than rust out, and her refusal to become inactive probably did help the mobility of her old joints. She swore by her bee pollen pills, which she got from a mail order house, guaranteed from genuine bee stingers. She took three a day to keep the arthritis suppressed.

Effie's activities revolved primarily around the Union Congregational Church and her neighbors. She was a mainstay of the Women's Guild of the church, and she also worked with the Youth Group. The church members were mostly older people. It wasn't easy to attract the younger people who were more interested in worldly activities, and who didn't worry much about their souls until considerably later in life. The church ministers were young, bright, and attractive, but usually stayed only until the opportunity came along for a bigger, wealthier, and less isolated congregation. Not infrequently the minister was a temporary practicing senior student from the venerable and respected Bangor Theological Seminary. All the ministers sought Effie's advice and used her vast knowledge of the people and the land because she had lived there and had been an important part of the community since the 19th century.

The Women's Guild raised impressive sums of money to support the church, especially in the summer when there were more people around. The women held baked goods and craft sales, used book and yard sales, fish chowder and baked bean suppers. Effie's doughnuts were widely considered to be far superior to Dunkin' Donuts or other commercial types and always were the first to sell out at the bake sales, as were her brownies, apple and blueberry pies, not to mention her strawberry-rhubarb preserves, and mustard pickles. She knitted sweaters, mittens, pillow covers, and made afghans and quilts for the popular craft sales.

Every Sunday she brought a nice dinner to a crippled shut-in neighbor. Every noontime during the week a friend came over to have lunch and watch their favorite television soap opera, "The Young and The Restless," which they referred to as "The Old and The Listless." Effie kept right up with the goings on in the world. She read the *Bangor Daily News* and watched the television news regularly. Her favorite was the "McNeil/Lehrer News Hour" because they asked such sensible and probing questions in their interviews with prominent newsmakers and authorities.

One day Effie noticed a little blood coming from her intestines, which prompted a visit to Ken Bunting, her friend and family doctor. Dr. Bunting examined her and said that he could feel a growth inside her rectum. He called Dr. Harry Byrd, who was 150 miles away at the closest hospital equipped to manage an extensive problem in such an elderly patient. While he listened to Bunting's description of the problem, Byrd felt discouraged about the prospect of treating a cancer of the rectum in a ninety-three-year-old lady. The usual treatment would be removal of the rectum and a permanent colostomy, but maybe they could settle for local removal and radiation treatments. This would pose additional problems because anybody, especially an old lady, would find it too difficult to travel 300 miles round trip from home to the hospital every day, except weekends, for six weeks to have the treatments. Perhaps they would just have to settle for localized removal of the cancer, which wouldn't give much chance for cure, but then how long does a ninety-three-year old expect to live, anyway? Byrd knew that

Bunting was an experienced, well-trained practitioner, and that his described findings would be reliable, so they arranged for Effie Haskell to enter the hospital directly the next day for studies and treatment.

Harry Byrd went to Effie's hospital room that next afternoon and found her son, pretty old himself at age seventy-two, anxiously sitting in the chair beside his mother's bed. If he was old, she was ancient at ninety-three, sitting up in the bed as perky and cheerful as could be, working on a cable-knit, blue sweater. She was a slim woman with twinkling eyes and smile lines radiating outward from their lateral corners.

"Is this problem serious?" the son asked.

"Just being ninety-three years old is serious," Byrd responded. They discussed the problem, and Effie told Byrd that she was ready for whatever needed to be done.

"I don't mind dying, and I am prepared for it. What bothers me is what I have to go through to get there."

He thought about the numerous other old Maine ladies he had taken care of who had similar impressive attitudes. They characteristically told him their complaint, and he figured out the problem. Then, he explained the findings to them and advised treatment, which they accepted. He did what was necessary, they got well, thanked him, and went home. This was, however, a different, tougher problem.

Byrd examined Effie and was perplexed to find that he couldn't feel anything abnormal in her rectum despite what reliable Ken Bunting had told him. He called in Daniel Harrier, the gastroenterologist, who arranged to do a colonoscopy, which might be described as a trip through the large bowel with gun and camera, starting at the bottom with a long flexible tube and working up. The gun is an electrocautery unit to remove or sample abnormal tissue, and the camera is an ingenious device to record the findings of Harrier's eyeball. After the bowel had been thoroughly cleansed with purgatives, an unpleasant process which Effie never complained about, Harrier did the colonoscopy. Not only did he solve the mystery, but he also cured the problem. There was, indeed, a growth the size of a golf ball, and instead of being fixed on the bowel wall, it was on a long string-like stalk that allowed it to slide up and down the bowel to different levels at different times. It was easily palpable at the time of Bunting's examination, but when Harry Byrd repeated the rectal examination, it had retracted upward and out of reach. The bleeding which Effie had noticed was caused by irritation of its surface or twisting of the stalk. Daniel Harrier cauterized and cut through the stalk at its base and removed the polypoid growth. Microscopic examination showed that it was not malignant.

Dr. Byrd rejoiced at the happy result of what he feared would be a terrible problem. He went to Effie's room. "You certainly look lovely today, Mrs. Haskell."

"Why, thank you, Doctor, and may God forgive you for being a liar," she responded.

"How are you feeling?" he asked.

"Rather languid," she said.

He explained the findings to her and her old son and told them that she could go home. The son said, "Well, there," and he exhaled audibly. Harry Byrd thought how many times here in Maine he had heard those two words, "Well, there" from patients' relatives when they had been told of a favorable outcome to their loved one's medical problem.

Effie's expression didn't change at all, but her eyes twinkled. "Won't they all be surprised when I walk into church on Sunday."

Indeed, they would be, Byrd thought, for everyone in Eastport knew that she had gone off to the hospital with trouble and wondered if she would survive it. In the small towns of Maine, and no doubt elsewhere in the country, everybody is saddened when one of their members has trouble, especially such a beloved person as Effie, and they rejoice when good things happen. This is unlike bigger cities where people seem to be clambering over the backs of everyone else to get ahead in the world and are unconcerned about the troubles of others.

As it turned out, there was one hitch in an otherwise happy outcome. When the Medicare representatives reviewed Effie's record, it was decided that hers was an unnecessary hospitalization. She could have been studied and treated at much less expense as an outpatient. There is entirely too much wastage of government funds by this sort of thing, and she was responsible for paying the hospital bill herself. Byrd appealed the decision on the basis that it was initially believed in good faith that the patient had rectal cancer. Not only that, but it was unfair to expect a ninety-three-year- old lady who lived 150 miles from the hospital to travel back and forth for outpatient studies and treatment. The appeal was rejected because of physician error and because the patient's age and distance of her home from the hospital were social problems, not medical ones. Harry Byrd felt as though his patient was being penalized for not having rectal cancer, a strange sort of situation, but then, he thought, life was becoming stranger and stranger all the time.

The Survivor

It seems that there are an endless number of older Maine ladies who have experienced sometimes happy, but often sad, long years of life and just accept with remarkable equanimity whatever life has in store for them. They are often survivors of bad marriages or widowhood and live with or without their men, have raised their families, even sometimes their children's families, the best way they could, always striving to produce honest, hardworking, God-fearing citizens. These older ladies are the backbone of Maine's social structure.

Sara Beal was one of those ladies. She had descended from an impressed English seaman who had survived a shipwreck before the Revolutionary War and decided to stay right there on the Maine coast where he was washed ashore, half dead. Sara trained to be a school teacher at Castine Normal School before it was converted to the Maine Maritime Academy. She married Josiah Beal, a young, hardworking fisherman, and they built their home at

Spruce Harbor where she lived most of her life. Sara bore Josiah two sons who were still young when their father was lost in a storm at sea. She grieved for her beloved husband, but accepted her lot and settled down to finish raising the boys alone, while continuing to teach school. One of the boys became the captain and owner of a seiner. The other managed and later purchased a lobster pound in nearby Ketch Cove.

Sara had retired from teaching and was age seventy when Harry Byrd had the good fortune to meet her. She had become pale despite frequent exposure to the sun and wind, had lost some weight, and tired easily. Her family doctor, Jonathan Partridge of Machias, found that she was anemic, and it was the type of anemia due to chronic blood loss. Sara hadn't noticed the blood because it was so slight, but there was a steady trickle of blood from a growth in the right side of her large bowel, and the growth, which was surely malignant, could be clearly seen on special x-ray studies.

When they first met in his office, Byrd looked at her across his old oak desk, which had become faded by the sun that streamed in his window. He saw a slim, simply dressed, pale woman who looked considerably younger than he had expected. Her long, grey hair was drawn back in a bun. With her hands relaxed in her lap, she sat quite composed in his red leather armchair and looked back at him steadily through calm, clear blue eyes. They talked for a while, and Byrd explained the problem to her with diagrams, then told her what needed to be done as well as the risks involved. Sara clearly understood the problem and wanted to know what the chances were for cure. Byrd said it was fifty percent, maybe better or maybe worse, depending on the findings at the operation. After more discussion and explanation about what she would experience and what everybody involved in her care would be doing, Sara was admitted to the hospital. The right half of her large intestine was removed, and the remaining divided ends of the bowel were connected together. Byrd removed that much to get well around the cancer and the lymph nodes which drained it. One can get along fine with little or even no large intestine. Byrd had a good feeling about her future, not only for the long term, because the cancer appeared to be confined to the intestine without spread to the lymph nodes or beyond, but also for the short term, because these older ladies almost always did better and recovered faster than anybody else, for some reason. He thought, perhaps, it was because of their philosophy of just accepting whatever came along and doing what had to be done, or because they were proven tough survivors beneath their fragile and delicate-appearing surface.

During the next week in the hospital Sara Beal and Harry Byrd became friends, something that almost always happened with Harry's patients. A bond developed between them that could be considered a form of love. Maybe this was one of the reasons he had never been sued. People can sense what their doctor's feelings and attitudes toward them are, whether or not the doctor really cares deeply about them as highly complex individuals, and how much the doctor gives of himself to help get them back to health. Byrd was a great worrier, and he was certain that worrying about patients helped, even though it took its toll on the worrier.

The worrier keeps thinking about the various possible things that can go wrong and finds those little, early, subtle indications of impending trouble so that corrective changes can be made before the trouble gets a jump on the patient. It turned out with Sara that Byrd didn't need to worry as much as usual. She had few complaints and no complications. During his daily or twice daily visits, he listened to her observations about life. A person can, of course, learn a lot by taking time to listen and among other things, he learned her formula for growing old gracefully:

1. Get dressed every day.
2. Eat three times a day.
3. Go out in the fresh air at least several times a week.
4. Grow something.
5. Read a book every two or three weeks.
6. Make yourself an expert on some subject.
7. Have company - invite someone in at least once a week.
8. Make new friends, preferably younger than yourself.
9. Do a thoughtful deed for another person at least once a week.
10. Never forget the importance of smiles and laughter. A sense of humor is a terrible thing to lose.

Harry Byrd wasn't sure if this formula was original to Sara, but he carefully recorded the formula for future reference, even though he figured he probably wouldn't last long enough to grow old gracefully himself. He did have a suggestion for Sara about how to become an expert on a subject. He had learned by observing some professors at medical school that you just talked about the subject all the time and then, whenever the subject came up, everyone, like Pavlov's dogs by reflex, thought of your name and asked for your opinion on the subject.

Sara went home to Spruce Harbor on schedule and came back as planned for a follow up visit four weeks later. She had regained considerable strength as well as the lost pounds. The pallor had gone, and her eyes were just as clear blue and steady as ever. The plan was to continue the customary regular checkups every six months or so. However, Sara never came back, and Byrd began to worry about why she hadn't kept her appointments. Customarily, he read the obituaries every morning in the *Bangor Daily News* to see if he knew anyone in there, including himself, and he had never seen Sara Beal's name listed. The bond between them had been broken until, as it turned out, several years later.

One bright summer morning during their vacation, Byrd and his wife set out early for a ride in their Buick Skylark along the Maine coast. You can drive more than a hundred miles over coastal U.S. Route 1 from Bucksport to Calais, Maine without hardly ever seeing the ocean you are driving along, with the notable exception of Sullivan Harbor. The coast is jagged and irregular with innumerable peninsulas, necks, points, bays, coves, and harbors. That explains why Maine's border with the sea is about 3,000 miles long if you walked along it, which you can't do because it is so rugged. It also explains why the rum-runners enjoyed considerable success bringing their contraband in from Canada during prohibition. In fact, one secluded spot tucked away near Eastport is appropriately named "Gin Cove." To really see the coast, it is necessary to drive quite a few miles down one of the many roads that go off to the east from U.S. Route 1. It would take about a year to go down and back on all those roads and see the entire coast from Kittery to Calais.

Harry and Avis drove through desolate stretches of Washington County with the vast blueberry barrens, fringed by scrubby fir trees and alders stretching to the horizon on both sides of Route 1. The fields were deep green, splashed with tinges of blue, since this was blueberry harvest time. Small and large granite boulders were scattered on the fields. In spring the barrens are black when they are burnt over to promote the growth of the low-bush wild fruit, then white with blossoms in early summer. In the fall they are colored brilliant red by the frost. Groups of bent-over workers were fanned out across the fields, raking blueberries or clustered around the winnowing machines that separated their blueberries from leaves, choke cherries, and other debris.

When Harry Byrd had first moved to Maine from Boston, which was one of the smartest things he ever did, he heard people talking about the blueberry barrens. Like a naive person "from away," and being of a romantic turn of mind, he had the foolish idea that they were referring to blueberry barons, somewhat akin to lumber barons. He pictured the barons as powerful landowners with swagger sticks, who drove around their fields in Land Rovers and wore pith helmets and jodhpurs while overseeing the backbreaking work of migrant Mic Mac Indians and school children who were paid near slave wages by the barons. In time Byrd had figured out the true blueberry situation and realized he was wrong except for the wages part.

When Byrd and Avis finally reached the Washington County seat of Machias, they stopped to eat their box lunch beside Bad Little Falls, where the Machias River tumbles down through a rocky gorge to join the ocean. They then turned back onto U.S. Route 1, and Avis agreed to take a ride down one of the side roads to the coast. Harry turned off at the sign "Spruce Harbor" with an arrow pointing east. He had an ulterior motive for taking this particular road because he wanted to find out what he could about Sara Beal. They drove for about twenty minutes. When they came to a cemetery about a mile or so before the harbor, Harry decided to stop there to look around. It would be embarrassing for all concerned if he inquired in the village and found that Sara had passed on. Her death might have been recorded in the *Ellsworth American*, but not the *Bangor Daily News*.

All the granite headstones in the graveyard faced the sea. Some of the inscriptions dated back to the eighteenth century. Wild blueberries grew in clumps all over the cemetery. Harry noted that many of the people buried there had lived into their seventies and eighties, but quite a few had died in the prime of life. Some markers simply recorded the passing of men who were lost at sea. There were a surprisingly large number of tiny headstones, marking the graves of infants and small children. Harry wondered how many could have been saved had they not been born before the development of vaccines for diphtheria, smallpox, measles, or whooping cough, and how many had died from diseases such as pneumonia, meningitis, or streptococcal infection before the antibiotic era. Even a relatively simple gastroenteritis could have been fatal to an infant without the availability of intravenous fluids to correct dehydration.

He found the Beal family plot and a headstone, arched at the top, with the inscription chiseled in the granite:

JOSIAH BEAL

1881-1919

LOST AT SEA

SARA BEAL

HIS WIFE

1884-

Harry was greatly relieved to see that although the gravesite was ready, Sara was not. He walked back to rejoin Avis at the roadside where she preferred to wait because of her aversion to cemeteries. On the way he picked a handful of blueberries, but when he thought of what was nourishing their roots beneath the ground in the graves, he couldn't eat them. He realized that was a foolish thought, but couldn't eat those blueberries anyway and threw them away. They drove into the village of Spruce Harbor, and Harry confidently asked at the general store where he might find Sara Beal. The storekeeper pointed through the window to a square, two-story clapboard house, neatly painted green on the upper half and white on the lower. It overlooked the harbor on the opposite side from where they were, near the wharf of the lobstermen's co-op. The harbor itself was oval-shaped and looked as if some powerful force had carved it, which in truth it had, from the granite that rose around its circumference. A short distance outside the narrow entrance of the harbor lay a strategically located island of rock covered with fir trees that barely hung on to the granite edges by their shallow roots. The island guarded the harbor entrance and broke the heavy Atlantic swells rolling in behind it. In fact, it was on this island that the ship carrying Sara Beal's seaman ancestor had been wrecked, though all her spars and timbers had long since disappeared. Spruce Harbor was, and still is, a commercial fishing village, and the fishermen subtly discourage visits by the summer pleasure yachts that cruise Maine's coast. If a yawl or cabin cruiser puts into the harbor, the yachtsmen are politely directed to guest moorings that are all at the back of the harbor. It just so happens that when the tide goes out, there is no water back there, so the expensive pleasure crafts get hung up and have to wait for the next high tide before they can be refloated and leave. As a result, not many pleasure crafts are to be seen in Spruce Harbor, unless of course, a coastal fog settles in pretty good, which it sometimes does, especially in the summer.

Harry Byrd drove around the dirt road that skirted the harbor, past fishermen's homes perched on the granite with stacks of lobster pots, buoys, and rope neatly piled outside. He pulled up beside Sara Beal's house. Harry and Avis both got out and knocked with the brass door knocker. Sara came to the door herself, for she still lived alone. Obviously, she had continued to grow old gracefully. She appeared to be in good flesh and good health and was pleased to see Harry and Avis, whom she hadn't met before. They must come in and visit, she insisted.

In the sitting room a large picture window overlooked the harbor below. Sara brought out her grandmother's English bone china and steeped some Formosa Oolong in the teapot. As Sara covered the pot with an embroidered tea cozy to keep it hot, Harry recalled the only other tea cozy he had ever seen was a wedding present, which he and Avis had never used. Sara served the tea with Scottish shortbread, while they talked. She explained that she had been fine right along since the surgery and didn't come back simply because if the cancer ever did recur, she didn't see that there was much anybody could do about it anyway at that point, so why bother. She had faith that it wouldn't come back, and in truth, it actually never did, then, or later. Byrd couldn't argue too hard against that point of view because if it had come back, he would have done a whole lot of things that wouldn't have really changed the basic situation much. On the other hand, periodic inspections of the remaining large bowel not infrequently turn up a newly developing precursor of another independent malignancy that could be removed without surgery, thus preventing future trouble. Sara smiled as she reminded Harry that she had already lived more than eighty years.

He did suggest that while she continued to grow old gracefully, she might include him in one of her rules, specifically the one about doing thoughtful deeds for others. Perhaps, she could drop a short note every year to let him know how she was faring. It would make him feel good to know his efforts were worthwhile. Sara agreed that made good sense. She talked about her sons, their children, and children's children. She also talked about life at Spruce Harbor and how it was sad that so many young people found it too hard a life trying to earn a living from the sea. Perhaps, they were not as tough as their forebears or looked at life differently. Many had gone off to Connecticut to work in the aircraft factories or to sew shoes in the shoe factories. It seemed to her that Maine's biggest export must be young people and not potatoes or timber! Byrd looked past her shoulder and through the big window. Shining in the late afternoon sun, the harbor was filled with graceful lobster boats with their classic sweet shear, tugging gently on their big, pink, plastic mooring balls. Not everybody could have moved out, he thought, because there was hardly any room for additional boats.

They bade Sara goodbye, and on the long drive home Avis said that she understood why he was so fond of the woman who was a survivor, just like her shipwrecked ancestor. They never saw Sara Beal again, but years later on another trip, Byrd stopped at Spruce Harbor cemetery on the way into the village. This time he knew what he would find.

JOSIAH BEAL

1881-1919

LOST AT SEA

SARA BEAL

HIS WIFE

1884-1972

"Eighty-eight years," he said aloud to himself. He deeply inhaled the clear salt air and looked at the headstones facing the sea in the silent graveyard. Harry knew that his life had been enriched by Sara Beal.